Full o' Beans!

Secrets to Transforming Your Health and
Life with a Whole-Food, Plant-Based Diet

HEIDI JENNINGS

Note from the Author

The information contained in this book is based around my personal study and experience of following a plant-based diet and forms the foundation of my coaching practice.

All efforts have been made to credit relevant sources of information.

Any decisions regarding prescription medication should be discussed with your doctor.

Real names have been used for case studies in Chapter Nine and for all testimonials. Where references have been made to other clients within the book, names have been changed to protect their privacy.

Testimonials

"When I first contacted Heidi, I was low on energy, feeling out of sorts and had a few kilos to lose. Within the first couple of weeks, I noticed my eyes were clearer, my stress levels had reduced, bloating was gone, and I was feeling much more energetic. I started to lose some weight and felt my jeans getting looser. The meal plans worked well for me and I enjoyed the variety of tasty foods. They were easy to stick to and gave me the fuel I needed to improve my energy levels. After six weeks, I felt so much better. I did encounter an emotional hurdle towards the end of the programme but because I was feeling stronger physically and mentally, I felt confident I could navigate my way through it. I'm so glad I completed the programme and am back to feeling like myself again!"

Treana, 60s

"I had suffered a few knocks over the past few years and wanted to feel better physically and mentally. I was experiencing some anxiety and depression and I knew it was partly because I was eating food that wasn't good for me. I wanted to lose some weight, address some gut issues, and just feel good again. I needed a plan to follow that would work! After a short period of time on Heidi's programme I started to feel a lot better. I got into a good sleep routine and started to experience more energy during the day. I enjoyed the variety of food on the meal plans and found them easy to follow. I started losing some excess weight and my moods became a lot more balanced. Because of this I was able to deal with stressful situations more calmly. This has been a lifestyle change for me and I feel so much better for it. Heidi's programme was just the thing I needed to get my health back on track."

Simon, 50s

"After six weeks of coaching, I had lost 3kg, which was quite impressive as I had some pretty big meals on a few of the days! I found the meal plans and support fantastic. I appreciated Heidi's advice and I liked the holistic approach in particular. I feel like I have found the way I would like to eat and live my life. I no longer crave bread, sweets and creamy lattes! Also, I am no longer worried about calorie restriction, which I feel is a real positive. In fact, I think I am consuming a lot more calories than I would have previously – and I still lost weight! It is much easier for me to not drink wine during the week, so I have also knocked out that habit. Other than just focusing on weight loss, I have made some positive changes that have become a real lifestyle change for the long term."

Shelley, 40s

"My main issues were high cholesterol, osteo-arthritic pain, menopausal hot flushes which meant I was on Hormone Replacement Therapy (HRT) medication, weight gain and anxiety. Heidi explained that my alcohol intake was working against me in all areas of my health. She encouraged me to lower my intake during the week, which I was able to do, and once I did that, in combination with following the meal plans, I noticed my problems were starting to lessen and resolve. My cholesterol came down to within the normal range, I came off my HRT medication because the hot flushes reduced, I was able to lower my anxiety medication, and I started to lose weight. I had to have an operation at the end of the programme, so while I am still in some pain, I now understand how reducing inflammatory foods and alcohol in my diet helps to lessen pain in the body.

It was great to experience first-hand how a plant-based lifestyle can start to heal all kinds of health conditions, and I was pleased with my progress in just six weeks. I am looking forward to continuing with this lifestyle and am confident that my body and health will continue to reap the benefits."

Anne, 50s

"When I first approached Heidi, I wasn't taking good care of myself. I was eating too much comfort food which left me feeling low on energy. At first, I was apprehensive about committing to the programme because I was worried about how it would fit in with family life, but I decided it was time to prioritise my health, and I'm so glad I did.

The meals on this plan are easy to cook and work in with family eating different things. They are also delicious, and there is plenty of food. Many of the recipes will become life-time favourites, I'm sure.

Within the first week of doing the programme, I noticed a vast improvement in my energy levels and mood over the course of the day (no more afternoon slump or after dinner cravings) and this continued throughout. Over the six weeks I also noticed a decrease in headaches and those little niggling aches and pains I often experienced day-to-day that can really zap your energy and leave you feeling irritable.

I really admire the way Heidi incorporates an holistic approach into her coaching. Having done a lot of work and study relating to emotional and mental health in recent years, I believe that addressing the whole person is the key to long-term success. Heidi is really easy to talk to and is very good at helping you see the positive side of things.

Doing this programme has fast-tracked my plant-based eating journey. I've come out the other side feeling I can continue on this path to better health with confidence. Thank you so much Heidi!"

Natasha, 40s

For Mum and Dad, who taught me the importance of good health and a positive attitude, and continue to walk the talk every day.

And for you, my reader, who has picked up this book because you know there's more waiting for you.

Welcome to your wonderful new way of life.

First published by Ultimate World Publishing 2022
Copyright © 2022 Heidi Jennings

ISBN

Paperback: 978-1-922828-34-7
Ebook: 978-1-922828-35-4

Heidi Jennings has asserted her rights under the Copyright, Designs and Patents Act 1988 to be identified as the author of this work. The information in this book is based on the author's experiences and opinions. The publisher specifically disclaims responsibility for any adverse consequences which may result from use of the information contained herein. Permission to use information has been sought by the author. Any breaches will be rectified in further editions of the book.

All rights reserved. No part of this publication may be reproduced, stored in or introduced into a retrieval system, or transmitted in any form, or by any means (electronic, mechanical, photocopying, recording or otherwise) without the prior written permission of the author. Any person who does any unauthorised act in relation to this publication may be liable to criminal prosecution and civil claims for damages. Enquiries should be made through the publisher.

Cover design: Ultimate World Publishing
Layout and typesetting: Ultimate World Publishing
Editor: Alex Floyd-Douglass

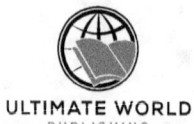

Ultimate World Publishing
Diamond Creek,
Victoria Australia 3089
www.writeabook.com.au

Contents

Note from the Author

Testimonials

Preface   1

Your Momentous Moment   3

Chapter One: Sowing the Seeds   7

Chapter Two: The Struggle of the SAD and Sick   23

Chapter Three: Meaty Milky Madness   39

Chapter Four: Nourishing Nutrition   57

Chapter Five: Potent Plants   79

Chapter Six: Setting the Scene   97

Chapter Seven: Practice is Power   113

Chapter Eight: Effortless for Everyone   135

Chapter Nine: Healthy and Happy   163

Chapter Ten: Delectable Dining   169

Recipes   178

Fabulously Full o' Beans!   199

About the Author   203

My Gifts to You   205

Acknowledgements   211

Further Reading & Viewing   213

Speaker Bio   215

Preface

After I finished writing my first book, *From Living Hell to Living Well*, I promised myself I would have a break and wait at least one year before embarking on the next one.

I promptly broke that promise within a matter of weeks, because in all honesty, I can't not write. Holding a pen and arranging words on paper came naturally to me from an early age, and it's always been something I am drawn to.

Now, while it's more efficient to touch type, I still find immense enjoyment in the process of telling a story that others might like to read – or even better, learn from.

My other love is health coaching. I have always had a strong interest in health and wellbeing, but the truth is, I've had to go through some rough times in my life when great health was not on my side. It was during those times that I developed the fundamental understanding that health is everything, and I am grateful that lesson appeared when it did.

It opened the door for me to discover all about the human body and the tools and strategies needed for optimal health and wellbeing – even better, it led me to the plant-based diet. What an incredible journey that has been, where I now have the privilege to share my experience and knowledge with my clients every single day and see them transition from down-and-out to on top of the world.

The fact I can combine my two loves of writing and health coaching into a little creation called a book is something that makes me indescribably happy. Becoming a published author for the second time? Well, that's nothing short of a dream come true.

And I know without a doubt that when you start to experience vibrant health and wellbeing for yourself, you too will soar and watch your own dreams come true.

Your Momentous Moment

Is there a time in your life that you look back on and realise – with hindsight – its profound significance? A moment that changed everything? A moment that, without it, you wonder where you'd be now?

Mine was the day I decided to pursue a plant-based diet. I had no clue how to go about it, what it would be like, and whether I could stick with it. All I knew was that I was very, very sick and that I would do anything to get better.

The motivation behind adopting a plant-based diet will be unique to each individual, yet there will always be a common theme. Whether it's for health, animal welfare or environmental reasons, the guiding light will always be because it just feels right.

It feels right to be healthy.

It feels right to protect animals and our precious environment.

And it certainly feels right to cling to hope that things can and will be better in the world.

At a time when so much threatens our survival and happiness, it's more important than ever to find something that provides a sense of security where we can thrive.

This desire isn't unique to humans; plants want this, too. Their ultimate mission is to put down roots in healthy soil, then reach their full potential by basking in sunlight and moisture. They harness the power of the natural elements so they can become full of colour and vibrancy and abundant in superpowers – otherwise known as nutrients.

Plants are a potent life force, and they exist on this earth to help other living beings reach their full potential, too. What an incredible gift they are to us!

Sadly, many of us won't reach anywhere near our full potential, because we don't understand how to nurture our physical, mental and emotional health. We exist, wither and die, because there are very few other options when we don't look after ourselves.

Then, there are those of us who will fulfil the life we were destined to lead, who will prosper and shine. It's not because we're better, or smarter, or fell from the lucky tree and hit every branch on the way down. It's because we do one very simple thing.

We appreciate the gifts provided by the earth, and we eat them. We allow their superpowers to infiltrate every muscle, organ and cell, where they create all kinds of magic to make our insides sing. Then, we repeat the process, day after day after day. What could be simpler than that?

I believe you have picked up this book because you want more out of life, and you're seeking to evolve. The desire to live our truth, fulfil our purpose and reach our incredible potential happens not only when we consistently work on improving ourselves physically and mentally, but also when we are willing to step beyond our comfort zone and try new things.

I would go so far as to say that being the best version of ourselves is not possible without optimal health, because health is what gives us the capacity to strive for and reach our dreams.

In my opinion, the best chance we have of enjoying the life we were given is by looking after the vessel we were born into, and as you are about to discover, the plant-based lifestyle is second-to-none for optimal health. Not only will this way of life supercharge the healing process and make you feel incredible, it will also give you the energy and desire to think outside the confines of the world you occupy and prompt you to ask yourself some of the bigger questions...

Who am I?

What do I want?

Who do I want to be?

Why am I here?

And when you start to answer those questions and follow where they lead, that's when the real magic happens.

When I first started writing this book, I had no intention of it being a sequel to *From Living Hell to Living Well*, but as I went along, I realised in many ways that it is. My first book is all about teaching you the fundamental principles to take charge of your health so that by the end, you have enough information to get the process underway – where I believe in this one, I take you through the concept of living well and catapult it into the stratosphere.

My main motivations behind writing this book can be summarised into two main points:

1. Provide easy-to-understand, straightforward information to those who are either curious about the plant-based lifestyle and need some guidance with how to go about it, or for those whose health is suffering, and are desperately searching for answers.
2. Highlight the incredible, life-changing sense of energy, vibrancy and wellbeing that occurs when plant-based foods form the basis of our diet.

My ultimate hope is that you will read this book and think, *"I can do this,"* and become inspired to experience this beautiful way of life for yourself.

And maybe, just maybe, this could be your momentous moment in time that changes everything for you.

CHAPTER ONE
Sowing the Seeds

Beginnings are never easy, and this particular one was no exception. It was January 2018, I was one month away from beginning my 40s, and this important milestone was not quite panning out the way I had imagined. I wasn't departing my 30s feeling on top of my game, reaping the rewards of a successful career, or planning a big birthday bash.

No. I was in the middle of the worst time of my life, experiencing a health crisis so bad that I spent most of my time in tears, depressed, and curled up on the couch, hoping to die in my sleep.

I was knee-deep in toxic heavy metal poisoning and topical steroid withdrawal (TSW), fighting a battle I desperately didn't want any part of. My daily list of symptoms was horrendous, from debilitating vertigo, eye floaters and night sweats, to itching and oozing skin so red and raw I looked like I had been burnt. I go into greater detail about my illness in my first book, *From Living Hell to Living Well*, but needless to say, I was as far from feeling *Full o' Beans!* as you can possibly get.

Searching for Answers

At a point of sheer desperation, I recall saying to my husband Steve, *"I don't think I want to cook meat anymore. I need to figure out a way to recover, and I think this might be it."*

"Okay, I'll support you with whatever you need to do," he'd replied.

And that was it. That was the day I stopped cooking and eating anything that came from an animal.

Because of my lifelong history with eczema, I had a very deep understanding of how food affected my body. Years earlier, fed up with being told to use steroid cream by my doctor and wanting to address the root cause of the problem, I worked alongside a naturopath to identify food and environmental allergens that were causing my red and itchy skin. I was able to remove a number of troublesome foods from my diet and watched in wonder as the eczema started to heal.

A few years later – as a result of toxic heavy metal poisoning – I developed eczema again which spread all over my face, neck and chest. Against my better judgement, I reverted back to steroid cream to reduce the redness and itch, not realising that cumulative steroid use over many years was about to result in the most horrific withdrawal when I stopped using the cream.

Sowing the Seeds

Now, I was in the midst of that withdrawal, and was in a very bad way, mentally and physically. My doctor, along with the rest of the medical establishment, refused to acknowledge TSW (a global problem and frankly, a disaster), and I realised this was a battle I was fighting alone. It was a dark and lonely place to be, and I spent months at a time wallowing in the misery of it all.

Simultaneously though, I was determined to get well again. Logic and common sense told me that if the body could heal the common cold or a graze on the skin innately, it could also heal deeper problems over time. I spent hours devouring all the information I could find on the subject of healing. Books, magazines, podcasts, YouTube clips – you name it, I read, watched, and listened to it.

In one particular podcast interview, I heard a piece of advice that stuck with me:

"Become an expert on yourself."

In other words, I had to become my own best expert about what worked for my body and what didn't, because no one else could do that for me. I had to develop trust in my body and understand what it was saying to me. That piece of advice served me very well and is now something I often share with my clients.

Thankfully, for the majority of the time I was sick, I was able to go out for walks. In fact, walking became my therapy, because it's the one thing that got me out of the house and allowed me to escape my miserable reality for a small chunk of time. A head wind was best, because the cool air calmed my flaring, red skin, drastically reduced the itch and allowed me to feel a small sense of relief – albeit briefly.

The symptoms of TSW include skin that is red, swollen, unbearably itchy, oozy and flaky, and this was occurring on my face, neck and chest for several months at a time. At my worst, I looked like a burn victim, and it made me very reluctant to be seen in public.

I became mostly housebound, but because I knew that walking helped me mentally, I would lace up my shoes, pull my cap over the open wounds on my scalp and forehead, and hope like hell I wouldn't bump into anyone I knew. I would set off with my earbuds in and listen to the most uplifting podcasts or audiobooks I could find.

They were usually stories about people who had suffered through dreadful health issues or had fought their way back from the brink of despair. These stories helped me realise I wasn't alone in my sadness and helplessness, and that perhaps, I too could recover. Some days I would walk for up to two hours at a time, just so I could listen to these incredible stories of people who had been where I was and had found health and happiness again.

The World of Plants

It was during these long walks that I learned as much as I could about the plant-based diet. As I had experienced first-hand the link between eczema and food, I wanted to delve further into the relationship between food and healing to see if I could speed up my recovery.

I wanted to know everything I could, and I found some excellent podcast channels that I returned to repeatedly. I felt like I had discovered this new and exciting world, and I knew I wanted to be part of it.

Sowing the Seeds

Tofu, chickpeas, nutritional yeast, jackfruit, cashew milk... The list was endless. I was fascinated about how all these new and wonderful foods could help me recover.

I started researching plant-based doctors and found an inspiring cache of professionals based in the USA who had been studying the field of plant-based nutrition for decades. They were able to provide compelling documentation and evidence about the sensational benefits of this lifestyle that I just couldn't ignore. An old school friend of mine is a devoted vegan, and she lent me a variety of books on the subject – which only added fuel to this fire of intrigue I had burning.

I remember the day I found the Instagram account of a young lady from the USA. I spent about three hours scrolling through her posts, watching video clips as she made incredible smoothie bowls and other plant-based goodies for her family. She too had once been chronically ill, desperate for night time to come so she could crawl into bed and escape her pain.

Now, she was a picture of health, with a beaming smile and glowing skin, thriving on plants. I was completely captivated and found myself getting joyfully lost in the #plantbased, #vegan and #plantoverprocessed hashtags.

I started researching plant-based recipes and venturing to the supermarket more often so I could search for these new and exciting ingredients. I would trawl the aisles, load up my trolley and couldn't wait to get home to start cooking. This new interest of mine was providing a much-needed beacon of hope during a very dark time.

I couldn't believe the taste sensations that were being created in my kitchen. I'm the first to admit that cooking is not my favourite past time, and I'd never put much thought or attention into cooking fancy meals. Now, I was excited to try these tantalising plant-based recipes, and boy, were they delicious. Much to my relief, Steve and the kids were enjoying them too, which took the pressure off me to cook two separate meals each night.

Even though I was the sickest I had ever been, this new way of life became a positive focus, and I started to feel confident that I could assist my body to heal if I just gave it the right food. I spent a lot of time in the kitchen trialling, taste-testing and coming up with all sorts of different concoctions. Instinctively I knew that I had found something that would help me become well again.

A Body in Harmony

By mid-2019, things were looking up. The symptoms from TSW had been at their worst between June 2017 and December 2018, and all I could do was take things one day at a time and look forward with longing to when things would be better. A very difficult part of TSW is not knowing when the symptoms will end.

I was involved with a global Facebook support group, where some people had been suffering for up to six years. It was pretty tough to know that I could be in for the long haul too. Thankfully, by the two-year mark, I was seeing dramatic improvements, even though my skin would continue to cycle through symptoms on and off for a further two years.

Throughout my darkest months and years, Steve would always remind me there was a bigger picture at play. He would tell me that we were in the middle of a huge lesson, and when we figured out how I could get better, we were going to be able to help a lot of people. As I started to recover, I thought about his words more and more.

What was the bigger picture here? What was the lesson? Could I find a purpose in all of this?

As it turned out, the answer was a resounding *yes*.

The more I followed the plant-based diet, the more I realised the incredible effects it was having on my physical and mental state. Physically, not only was my skin healing and the vertigo and eye floaters disappearing, I realised I just felt really *good* most of the time. I had consistent energy levels, was sleeping well, had no pain or discomfort, my tummy was flat, and my weight was stable.

Mentally, I noticed my thoughts were clear, I had great concentration and mental focus, and I felt happy. By happy, I mean very content – pretty much all of the time – aside from common life stressors that popped up occasionally. The best way to explain it was that I felt like my body and mind were humming and everything was working in harmony.

I knew without a doubt this was not a coincidence. The beautiful fresh, nutrient-dense foods I was eating all day, every day were contributing to this incredible state of wellbeing. Feeling so good after two years of hell was indescribable.

But, I needed more. I needed to know the nuts and bolts of *why*. Why was the plant-based diet so good? What was the reason for it all?

And, floating around in the back of my mind was the thought that if I was feeling like this, surely everyone else could, too! Maybe I could, after all, help a lot of people...

Learning the Ropes

One of the doctors I had been following, an American in his 80s named Dr T Thomas Campbell had written a book called *The China Study*. It was an intense read – more like a textbook – containing screeds of data he had gathered over decades studying the detrimental effects of animal protein on the Chinese population. The evidence from his studies was so compelling that he became someone I admired and respected in the area of plant-based living.

I became aware of a course he was offering through Cornell University in New York; a certificate in Plant-Based Nutrition studies. I signed up to his newsletter, and every now and then, I would open my email Inbox to another announcement about this course. In one particular newsletter, there was a banner along the top stating there was a 15% discount on the course if you registered within the next 48 hours.

I mentioned it to Steve, and how much I would like to do it. I reckoned that once I had more background knowledge about the plant-based diet, I could introduce it as an option to clients in our business. Up until this point, Steve had run our business solo. He had recently rebranded himself from a personal trainer to a holistic health coach, more accurately reflecting his skills and experience. I realised the potential of completing the course and how it could add another string to our bow.

"Okay," he'd said. "But if you're going to do it, I want you to make sure you actually use it."

What he meant was, if you're going to spend the money on this course, you better follow through with what you've promised!

I signed up immediately and couldn't wait to get started. As soon as the kids were off to school each morning, I would settle in front of my laptop, ready to soak up every word, furiously scribbling notebooks full of new wisdom.

The course was set out in a series of three modules, and at the end of each one, I felt regret that I was getting closer to the end – which sounds odd, but I was utterly absorbed in what I was doing and absolutely loved every single minute of it.

Learning about nutrition in society, diseases of affluence, environmental impacts, putting the plant-based lifestyle into practice and so much more was one of the most enjoyable learning experiences I've ever had. I can't say enough about studying a subject you are passionate about!

By the end, I felt confident that my first-hand experience, plus what I had learned in the course gave me enough knowledge to start helping others with their transition to a plant-based diet. I spent hours putting together a coaching manual, meal plans, grocery lists and recipes, set up a Facebook page and through our existing business channels, announced I was open for business.

Sharing the Love

The response was immediate and overwhelming. Within three days, I had four clients registered and I started to panic. Because I hadn't expected to get clients so soon, my manual and meal plans weren't complete. I had to spend a few days working non-stop to get everything ready. I won't lie – it was stressful, but at the same time, I was so excited to get started.

The results for my clients were instant. By instant, I mean within a week or two. By the end of six weeks, it was like talking with a brand-new person. Their chronic pain was gone. Their anxiety was gone. No more bloating. No more pesky hot flushes. Weight loss. Great sleep. The list went on and on. I knew I was onto something great.

At the same time, I was having a blast with my Facebook page and gathering followers. I started making short, 20-30 second videos showing how to make all sorts of meals, sweet treats, and smoothies, and setting them to punchy music. I wrote blog-type posts about anything and everything related to the plant-based lifestyle. I just loved it, and I realised that most of my audience had never seen anything like it before.

I'd get so many questions, such as:

"Where do I find coconut milk and cacao powder?"

"What is buckwheat?"

"I like the look of this, but where do I start?"

Right from the beginning, I had a steady stream of clients flooding in, and the same thing would happen every time. A client would come to me feeling fed up and stuck with their state of health, and by the end of the coaching programme, they were well on their way to feeling incredible. I started gathering testimonials from clients who were raving about our programme and saying it was life changing.

Within one year, I had worked with dozens of clients, written for a global digital magazine on the subject of health and wellbeing, had been invited to speak on stage and had just started writing our first book.

Six months later, our book was published and became an Amazon #1 bestseller in 23 categories, I was a regular columnist for a local foodie magazine, we were getting publicity for our business in newspapers and on national radio, and my writing was featured on several renowned global digital publishing platforms. I was on one heck of a ride and loving every moment of it.

Today, I love nothing more than to talk and write about the plant-based lifestyle. I simply love working with my clients, showing them how simple and straightforward it is to transition over to plant-based eating, and the reward that comes from seeing them start to thrive is like nothing else I've ever experienced.

Plant-Based vs Vegan

Sometimes I get asked why I call myself 'plant-based' and not 'vegan'. The simple answer is that plant-based feels like a better fit for me.

Firstly, you may be wondering what 'plant-based' actually means. Essentially, a whole-food, plant-based (WFPB) diet is one that revolves around plant-based foods, specifically fruits, vegetables, wholegrains, legumes, nuts, seeds and healthy fats. A plant-based diet does not include any animal products, such as meat, fish, dairy products or eggs, and there are very few processed and packaged foods or oils.

Plant-based indicates that the majority of my diet consists of plants (approximately 95% in my case), but there is a small allowance for non-plant-based foods occasionally, or what I like to refer to as 'wriggle room'.

For example, if my kids are eating a burger or an ice cream and they offer me a bite, sometimes I might say yes. If I'm out for dinner or at a friend's house and there's little in the way of plant-based options available, I may have a little bit of meat.

A vegan is generally far stricter and won't eat any animal products, ever. I admire people who call themselves 'vegan' if they follow a strict diet and have a strong commitment to animal or environmental welfare. Don't get me wrong; I think veganism is extremely important in protecting animals and the environment, but if I'm completely honest, health was my top consideration when it came to changing the way I ate.

People can also call themselves vegan and exist on junk food. You can drink gallons of coke and eat *Oreo* cookies and French fries all day every day and call yourself a vegan, but it doesn't mean it's healthy.

At a rough guess, I'd say that Steve and our two kids are 80% plant-based. I don't cook meat anymore, but from time to time Steve will buy a rotisserie chicken or cook some sausages on the barbeque. I do my best at home to give my kids a healthy, balanced diet through mostly plant-based foods, but when they are with friends or extended family, I am relaxed about what they eat.

I have a deep respect for any parent who manages to keep their family on a strict plant-based or vegan diet, but for me, that would involve a level of stress I'm not prepared to take on! I hope that while they are young, I can instil some good habits into my kids that they will fall back on as adults, but I'm not going to get tied up in knots about it. I do my best, and that's good enough for me.

Do I have days when I don't stick to a plan and skip lunch because I'm busy, or shove a frozen pizza in the oven for the kids at 6pm?

Yes, I do, but I don't worry too much about that. I accept those days for what they are, know that they are part of life from time to time, and simply just move on.

In my view, plant-based living should be about eating great, wholesome food and experiencing fabulous health and wellbeing – while at the same time being able to kick back and relax with some treats occasionally. This is the true definition of balance and will provide a lifestyle that can be easily sustained over the long term.

Whether you want to call yourself vegan and be very strict, or plant-based and allow yourself some space to cheat every once in a while, is completely up to you. The only rule is that you do what feels right.

My Promise to You

Before we get into the exciting, nitty gritty of the what, why and how of the plant-based diet, I want to make you a promise.

Assuming you do not have a terminal illness, incredible things start to happen when you follow a plant-based diet, and here are just a few:

- Your body starts to heal from the inside out, to the point where you start to remember what it's like to feel good, every day.
- Your mind becomes clear, and you find yourself sailing through the day without the emotional peaks and troughs you may have grown used to.
- The functions of your body start to recalibrate and perform exactly as and when they should.

- Excess kilograms fall off and you reach a weight that is right for you.
- Your joints and limbs carry you wherever you need to go with flow and ease.
- You realise your coping mechanisms for stressful situations have strengthened.
- You start to experience a state of vibrant health and wellbeing that you may have forgotten (or never knew) even existed.
- The future looks bright, even when you have difficult days.
- You realise you can do things you could never do before.
- You experience a sense of contentment that money just can't buy.

In a nutshell, life becomes extraordinary, enjoyable and effortless.

Our bodies communicate with us constantly, and it's so important that we learn to listen to what they are saying. When we can do that, and start taking responsibility for how we treat them, we are rewarded with the magic of vibrant health. This results in a beautiful freedom to live our lives in the best way we can.

And there's simply nothing better than that.

Digging up the Dirt

On a scale of 0-10, where 0 is 'dreadful' and 10 is 'incredible', where do you currently sit with regard to your overall state of health and wellbeing? And why?

_____

_____

_____

_____

_____

_____

_____

_____

_____

_____

_____

_____

_____

_____

CHAPTER TWO
The Struggle of the SAD and Sick

It's been over four years since I adopted a WFPB diet, and in that time, I've realised just how easy and straightforward it is, for both myself and the people I work with. But I also know that the vast majority of the world's population don't eat this way, and the thought of doing so is either very unappealing, or somewhat daunting.

Why is this? Surely eating well is a natural and instinctive thing to do?

Biologically, yes, it is but somehow, we have lost our way when it comes to following our instincts and nourishing our bodies.

Have you heard of the Standard American Diet? It's abbreviated to the SAD for a very good reason. This is the diet most of the western world follows, and it's having very serious (and sad) consequences.

A typical day of eating on the SAD looks something like this:

Coffee with sugar-coated cereal and milk for breakfast, coffee and a buttered scone for morning tea, a chicken salad sandwich with margarine and drowned in mayonnaise on white or brown bread for lunch, coffee and a couple of chocolate biscuits for afternoon tea, lasagne laden with cheesy sauce for dinner washed down with a glass of wine or beer, and a cup of tea with another couple of chocolate biscuits before bed.

How many of those foods and drinks are natural, fresh and full of nutrition? None of them! All are heavily processed and packed with calories, fat, sugar and salt. Perhaps our bodies could manage this onslaught on the odd occasion, but people are eating this way *every single day.*

Think about where you sit on that scale of 0-10 with your overall state of health.

In my experience, most of my clients are below a five when they first come to see me, and the vast majority of them are following the SAD. By the end of my coaching programme, they are usually an eight or above, and the SAD has been banished to a distant memory. Coincidence? I think not.

If you've read my first book, you'll know that 7 out of 10 of our leading causes of death are related to nutrition.[1]

---

[1] *(April 27, 2016, U.S. Centers for Disease Control and Prevention (CDC), at: http://www.cdc.gov/nchs/fastats/leading-causes-of-death.htm)*

The Struggle of the SAD and Sick

In other words, 70% of the most common ways to die are a direct result of the stuff we are putting in our mouths. 70%! If that's not a sad state of affairs, I don't know what is.

We know that Americans have a reputation for super-sized portions and the bellies to match, but we can't just point the finger at them. A large proportion of the western world has followed suit – to the point where globally, 52% of all adults were found to be overweight or obese in 2021, and worldwide, obesity rates tripled since 1975. (*World Health Organisation, Obesity and Overweight, 9 June 2021*)

These are staggering statistics that equate to *billions* of people who are staring down the barrel of an early death.

Interestingly (or tragically in my view), the subject of nutrition has an incredibly low ranking in medical schools and receives barely any funding. In fact, there has been very little change in the way nutrition is taught in the past few decades, and it's not uncommon for a trainee doctor to receive only about 20 hours of training on the subject of nutrition over four years. Even then, the focus is on bio-medical factors, such as how macronutrients are metabolised in the body, not how nutrition plays a role in the prevention and treatment of disease. *(Thomas Campbell, Influencing Nutritional Practices: Training Healthcare Professionals, 2020)*

This is hardly surprising when we know that conventional medicine does not acknowledge the strong correlation between nutrition and health.

> *"As a physician, I am embarrassed by the lack of initiative and obstructionist policies of my own medical profession towards healthier lifestyles."*
>
> (Dr Caldwell Esselstyn)

Unless we bring more awareness to why our society has such a poor state of health, nothing will ever change and will only get worse, which as a parent and hopefully future grandparent, is concerning.

Fortunately, the growth of the plant-based movement is forging ahead, but relatively speaking, it's still in its infancy. Most of the western population is still chugging along on the SAD train, ignorantly unaware of the wreck that lies ahead.

So, what has gone so wrong? Why, as a society, have we deviated so far away from being fit and healthy beings? Is it because we're all just lazy, unmotivated and can't be bothered to do better?

To some degree, perhaps. But there are even bigger, deeper problems, and this chapter is dedicated to bringing awareness to what those problems are so we can make the choice to consciously step away from them and choose a healthier path.

The key issues outlined below are related to confusion, factors that influence our behaviour, paradigms, policy and politics, and our busy lifestyles.

Confusion

A key factor in our society's poor state of health is general confusion. People are perplexed about what should be a very simple and straightforward subject; how and what to eat for a healthy body.

If you take a good look around, there is plenty of evidence of this. Browse through a health and fitness magazine, and you will see an article about the benefits of high-fat diets. Then find a similar magazine from five years ago, and you'll read all about the virtues of eating low-fat.

Go to your local gym, and the personal trainers will explain why you should be doing high-intensity exercise to burn body fat. Then talk to a yoga guru, who will tell you all that stuff is overrated and what you really need to focus on is your breathing and alignment.

Or how about this one: *"Fruit is bad for you."*

What? Suddenly, after humans have survived and thrived on fruit for thousands of years, nature's candy is now the enemy?

High-carb or low-carb? Bananas or bacon? Feasting or fasting?

It goes on and on, and really, it's no wonder people don't know what they're supposed to be doing. The health and wellness industry is a melting pot of contradictory and confusing information, not helped in the slightest by the latest 'scientific studies' that shift the goalposts every five minutes.

A key thing to remember is that often the primary driver behind the health and wellness industry is profit. Trends, fads and the latest diet are very much about making the manufacturers and marketers rich, and very little to do with improving your health.

Influencing Factors

The way we eat is largely influenced by background factors that we don't think about much on a day-to-day basis but are actually very significant.

Full o' Beans!

We are all brought up with core belief systems that become ingrained in our subconscious from an early age. Think about some nutritional beliefs that may have been instilled in you from your parents and other family members.

Beliefs can stem from both words and actions. How did your biggest influencers talk about food and drink? Did they have a *'Who cares, you only live once'* attitude, or were they more restrained?

How did they act? Did they starve or stuff themselves? Did they have a couple of drinks then stop, or did they keep going until they were comatose on the couch?

Were they happy in their own skin, or did they grimace in the mirror while grabbing fat rolls around their middle?

The words and actions we are surrounded with as a young child are very powerful and deeply affect us – even if we're not consciously aware of them.

Now, think about the emotional factors that may have influenced you over the years. Were you rewarded for good behaviour with treats? Were you punished for bad behaviour by missing out on dinner?

Have you continued those patterns into your adult life, where you now indulge in junk food because you 'deserve it' after a hard day? Or do you punish yourself for over-indulging by starving yourself for the next two days?

Financial factors can also play a role. Could your family afford to indulge in luxuries which meant unhealthy treats were always available, or did your parents buy good quality, more expensive food? Did the food budget only just stretch to three basic meals per day, or mean that there was a reliance on cheap convenience foods with little nutritional value?

Think about the culture you were brought up in. Did socialising with family and friends revolve around tables full of food and drink where everybody tucked in to excess? Did your grandmother express her love for you by cooking roast dinners with all the trimmings and spoiling you with endless puddings and lollies?

All of these factors influence how we perceive and act around food from a young age and into adulthood, and much of it is subconscious behaviour which can continue for a lifetime – unless we consciously become aware of it and decide to make changes.

One of the main catalysts for change is a serious health issue which forces attention towards healthier habits. For me, that catalyst was eczema that continued to worsen throughout my 20s and 30s and demanded that I pay more attention to my diet. Then, it was my later experience with toxic heavy metal poisoning and TSW, where I delved further into nutrition to help me recover.

In many ways, I feel lucky these things happened while I was still relatively young. Many people can get away with a poor diet until health issues start to surface later in life, and by then, it can be very difficult to reverse a lifetime of unhealthy habits and behaviours.

That doesn't mean it's impossible though. All it takes is awareness, and a decision to change. 80% of making a change is based on mindset, and the other 20% is having the right tools, knowledge and support to guide you in the right direction.

Paradigms

In simple terms, a paradigm is a set of ideas or way of looking at something that can determine how things are studied and how the results are explained.

Our dominant nutritional paradigms have formed over time through scientific studies which are reported as the truth, while often ignoring other points of view. One such paradigm has contributed to a population of very sick people, and this has been coined by Dr T Colin Campbell as *"The local theory of disease."*

The local theory of disease is where doctors believe that there are very specific causes for very specific diseases. For example, lung cancer is caused by cancerous cells in the lung, which then must be treated by chemotherapy or removal of damaged tissue. There is no real consideration of the deeper reasons for why cells are becoming cancerous in the first place.

This is a 'reductionist' viewpoint, where the body is treated as a series of single parts in isolation from each other. Conventional medicine is still operating under the 'reductionist' or 'disease management' paradigm. A doctor will assess symptoms, use isolated treatments (such as removal of the diseased lung) and unnatural chemicals, and take a reactive approach to health.

This widespread viewpoint unfortunately has the consequence of discrediting other concepts.

"The best kept secret in medicine is that sometimes, given the right conditions, the body can actually heal itself. The body is a self-healing machine."

(Dr Michael Greger)

The Struggle of the SAD and Sick

Doctors who endorse the plant-based diet, such as Dr Campbell and Dr Michael Greger, take a 'wholistic' viewpoint, where the body is treated as a whole, and every part has a relationship with all other parts.

In our western world, every time someone visits their GP, the local theory of disease is applied. Medical interventions are ignoring the root causes of health problems, which means that symptoms are simply treated with medication and will often resurface.

The wholistic paradigm is where the importance of nutrition comes in. This approach is preventative rather than reactive, uses whole foods, investigates underlying causes for disease, and prefers systematic treatments. Unfortunately, this approach is still largely ignored within the medical establishment and is only applied by more alternative and holistic practitioners.

Globally, there are a few doctors who are doing the research and working diligently to show the impact of nutrition on health outcomes, but paradigm shift takes a long time and is a challenging process.

In the meantime, while we wait for change to happen, we can simply look around us for all the evidence we need that our current approach isn't working.

And what do we do when something isn't working? Do we keep doing the same thing over and over again and expect different results? No! We must do things differently.

Policy and Politics

Our government has a lot to do with what we eat. It is supposed to protect the interests of both industry and consumer, but the reality is that industry can exert a lot more power. The tactics used by influential industries go a long way to explaining why our natural instincts surrounding food have become warped and confused. Take a look below at just a few of the sneaky ways we are being deceived and manipulated.

Lobbying is where private interest groups attempt to influence decisions made by the government. For example, the meat, dairy, alcohol and junk food industries have many different lobbying groups who have plenty of money to spend on building close relationships with decision-makers, so they can essentially bribe them into giving them what they want. Health food lobby groups on the other hand lack the power and resources to fight against them.

Astroturfing or 'fake grass roots' is a deceptive practice where organisations employ online identities and fake pressure groups who appear to represent real people, but in actual fact are advocating for large corporations.

For example, when the State of New York proposed a soda tax in 2010, *Coca Cola* formed a group called "Americans Against Food Taxes" – where people were paid to publicly 'protest' against the tax.

Public Relations tactics also make up a massive part of lobbying. For example, when junk food companies co-opt scientific studies to publish 'research' in support of their product.

'Front groups' are formed to make it look like they are representing consumer interests but are actually funded by large industries. For example, the Beverage Institute for Health and Wellness was set up by *Coca Cola* under the guise of supporting nutrition research and education — while deflecting any notions that their products might be harmful.

These are just a few examples of deceptive practices used by the food and beverage industry to manipulate our eating habits, and fearmongering is a big part of it.

Busy Lifestyles

The information above provides some background understanding about why our society is in the middle of a train wreck health-wise. Yes, we are confused, we are impacted by subconscious beliefs that stem from our upbringing, doctors operate under a system of medicating rather than addressing the root cause of a problem, and the food and beverage industry are very sneaky and underhanded a lot of the time. These are all very real scenarios and go a long way to explaining why we're in such a mess.

But there's another contributing factor that can't be overlooked, and that is, in today's modern world, we are overscheduled, overworked and overtired. Our lives have become so busy that by default we have abandoned the fundamental principles that keep us healthy.

Using my clients as 'case studies' is a very useful way of explaining real-life examples, so let me tell you about Jane, a lady I worked with about six months ago.

Jane is 51 years old and works full-time as an accountant. Her job involves long hours, a demanding boss and little flexibility in terms of time off or working outside of the office. She is married and has three children: one away at university and two still living at home. Her husband also works full time and does a lot of domestic travel as part of his job, so he is away from home quite often.

Jane suffers from chronic back pain which is aggravated by sitting down for long periods of time. She has gained a lot of weight over the past few years which she attributes to a sedentary job, little time to exercise, and little desire to exercise anyway because of her sore back. Her doctor has prescribed pain killers in an effort to get on top of the pain. She has a constant feeling of lethargy and fatigue so drinks coffee throughout the day to keep her awake and focused at work.

She is frustrated by her kids, who she thinks are lazy and preoccupied with their iPhones, and she ends up doing the bulk of the household chores. She gets home from work at 5.30pm and the first thing she does is pour herself a glass of wine. She finds cooking a drag and relies a lot on convenience foods such as microwave meals and frozen pizza or throw-together meals such as nachos. Her kids are supposed to cook one night each per week, but Jane can't be bothered with the arguments that ensue if she mentions it, so she thinks it's easier just to do it herself.

By the time dinner is eaten, she is exhausted and wants to spend the rest of the night on the couch. Her kids retreat to their rooms to do homework and she feels bored and lonely, so she has another glass of wine. An hour or two later, still bored and feeling unfulfilled by Netflix, she has a cup of tea and brings a packet of Toffee Pops to the couch. It's not uncommon for her to have three or four biscuits in one sitting.

Before she knows it it's 11pm and time for bed. She finds sleep unrefreshing and more often than not, will hit the snooze button

The Struggle of the SAD and Sick

multiple times before getting out of bed in the morning. Then it's off to work, and the cycle repeats.

On the weekends, she spends her time running her kids to and from sports games, trying to fit in a catch-up with friends and family, and loves to get out in the garden – she loves gardening so much that she's prepared to put up with the back pain.

When I first met Jane, she got very emotional when telling me her story. She thought she might be suffering from depression because she felt constantly low, and that life was like Groundhog Day. She hated her job, felt underappreciated by her family and the only thing that brought her any joy was her garden. She said to me, *"There must be more to life than this."*

I see many clients like Jane, whose lifestyles and daily habits are creating serious health problems such as pain, depression, excess body fat and so on. These people might be doing their best to live a productive, healthy life but are falling short because they are too overwhelmed. Looking after their health ends up at the bottom of the priority list because there's too many other things to do.

In Jane's case, her late nights, alcohol and coffee intake, convenience foods and lack of exercise are resulting in poor health. As a result of poor health, she finds no enjoyment in life or her job. Because she feels no enjoyment, she has no motivation or desire to focus on getting healthy. Can you see how this becomes a vicious cycle?

"What's this got to do with a plant-based diet?" I hear you asking.

Well, a lot actually. Healthy nutrition is so fundamental to our overall state of wellbeing that what we eat or don't eat has flow-on effects to the rest of our life. In Jane's case, she was relying on junk foods that provide no nutritional value because she was too busy to think about eating properly. This created gut problems, mental health problems, liver problems, weight problems and sleep problems.

Everywhere you look, there's a Jane. Or a James. Working too hard, trying to fit too much in, not eating properly, drinking too much, and suffering the consequences. They are the epitome of the struggle with the SAD and sick.

Being busy is not necessarily a bad thing. The problem is busy-ness at the expense of good health. We must slow down, take a step back, and focus on our health first and foremost if we want to live long and happy lives.

If you feel like changing your eating and drinking habits is too big a task, or that you won't have support from your family and friends, or that you've got too much to deal with right now and will 'do it later', it's worth asking yourself some simple questions.

Can you afford not to change?

Are you prepared to face the consequences of your choices that will inevitably surface when you become sick?

Do you really want to live this way for the rest of your life?

Evidence of our global health crisis is all around us. Look at your friends, family members, neighbours and colleagues. I bet not a day goes by where someone you know isn't struggling with all manner of health issues. Or, perhaps that person is you?

The whole purpose of this book to show you it doesn't have to be this way. You can experience amazing health and wellbeing. You

The Struggle of the SAD and Sick

can become the best version of you. You can heal your body and mind and find your sparkle again.

A population of sick, stressed and unhappy people is avoidable, but realistically, it's going to take a really long time to see this on a grand scale. We can't control what other people do, but we can control our own actions and lead the way to becoming healthier individuals.

For this to happen, we absolutely must move away from the struggle of the SAD and sick and focus on the one key thing that will bless us with optimal health.

We must focus on the right nutrition.

Digging up the Dirt

Can you identify any factors mentioned in this chapter that have contributed to your eating or lifestyle habits? Are there any others? What are they and how have they impacted your current state of health?

_____

_____

_____

_____

_____

_____

_____

_____

_____

_____

_____

CHAPTER THREE
Meaty Milky Madness

Now we have a clearer picture of how we came to be on the destined-for-disaster SAD train – including your own personal contributing factors – it's time to take a closer look at the far-reaching impacts this way of life is having on our health and the world in which we live.

There tends to be a general lack of awareness (and lack of care) about the problems generated by our eating habits because they have become so ingrained and normalised. To some degree, it's a case of 'we don't know what we don't know' – although this excuse is starting to wear thin. Thanks to the glorious world wide web, we now have access to the evidence being introduced by forward-thinking doctors in the plant-based nutrition field. Without them doing the background work and presenting the results, I shudder to think where our world would be headed.

Understanding the effects of the SAD on the health and wellbeing of the human race and the environment is so important because it allows us to take a stand and find better ways of doing things. It empowers us to take control of our health – rather than leave it in the hands of a clearly flawed medical system that continues to ignore the strong link between nutrition and health.

It's obvious our modern eating habits aren't working well. I always find it fascinating to watch old video footage, say pre-90s, of crowds of people who pop up occasionally on television. It's very rare to see someone who is obese or even slightly overweight. Those were the days when Supersize Big Mac meals and all-you-can-eat buffets didn't exist.

Now, when you observe a large crowd or even those who walk past you on the street, more than half will be overweight.

The following quote perfectly sums up our collective mentality around health:

> *"Eating a vegetarian diet, exercising every day and meditating is considered radical. Allowing someone to slice your chest open and graft your leg veins into your heart is considered normal and conservative."*
>
> (Dr Dean Ornish)

Our society has become very confused about what is normal. Supersize Big Mac meals or going back for three large platefuls of food at a buffet is not normal eating behaviour, and yet we don't bat an eyelid. Triple bypass surgery on a diseased heart is not normal either, yet we've come to regard it as a common and acceptable life-saving procedure.

A lot of people don't care about what they're eating until a health crisis looms. A good doctor might warn about high cholesterol or lowering blood pressure by eating less red meat or drinking less alcohol, but because conventional medicine doesn't place enough emphasis on the correlation between food and health, people aren't being informed about how to eat *properly*.

So, that's what we're going to talk about here! Let's take a closer look at what the evidence says about some of our common, everyday foods and what they are doing to our health and the environment.

The China Study

The China Study is a long-term study carried out in the 70s and 80s by Dr T Colin Campbell (Cornell University) in partnership with researchers from Oxford University and the Chinese Academy of Preventative Medicine. This was the most comprehensive study ever undertaken on the relationship between diet and the risk of developing disease.

Prior to this, tests had been carried out on rats which showed that a diet high in animal-based protein promoted disease, whereas a diet high in plant foods had the opposite effect. Dr Campbell and his team set out to find out whether the same applied to humans.

As already mentioned, *The China Study* is a whopping great academic textbook full of data, facts and figures. If you love that kind of thing, I recommend you grab a copy from your local library and get stuck in. If you'd rather something a little easier to digest, read on as I summarise some of Dr Campbell's key findings in simple language, along with some key findings from other research.

China was chosen for the study because it had a large population, there was very little migration, the food production systems were localised, and the Chinese ate a diet high in plant-based foods. Even so, diet varied between populations in different geographical areas, and this study provided an opportunity to study the difference in disease rates between areas.

Over 6,000 adults were surveyed over a period of 20 years, using blood and urine samples, food samples, questionnaires and surveys regarding geographical factors. A significant finding was that a diet high in animal products was strongly associated with chronic, degenerative disease and higher blood cholesterol levels.

Below are some specific findings of *The China Study* as they relate to three of our top killers; cancer, heart disease and diabetes.

Cancer

There's a widespread belief that cancer is primarily initiated by chemical carcinogens. This has led to other potential causes (such as nutritional imbalances) getting ignored.

The China Study found that excess consumption of casein (a protein in cow's milk) was directly related to the development of pre-cancerous foci (tumour cells that can only be seen microscopically). This is because the biochemical response in the body from casein increases production of growth hormones and elevates the load of acid in the body. *(Dr T Colin Campbell, PhD, Nutrition & Gene Expression in Cancer Development, 2020)*

Interestingly, foci increased with higher levels of casein in the diet (above 10%) but reduced with lower levels of casein (below 10%), leading to the conclusion that dietary protein levels could effectively turn on or turn off early foci development.

Dr Campbell's research found that casein and other animal proteins were likely to be far more carcinogenic than any other herbicide, pesticide, noxious chemical or food additive.

Another significant finding of the study was that nutrition actually controls the genes involved in cancer development, even if the cancer is initiated by a carcinogen or viral activity, and can essentially halt and reverse cancer development in the initiation and promotion stages.[2]

His overall conclusion was that cancer could be prevented by a diet low in fat and animal protein, and higher in plant protein and carotenoids (colour components of vegetables).

In 1931, German physiologist and medical doctor, Otto Warburg, was awarded the Nobel Prize for his work showing that an acidic cellular and circulatory system in the body could cause cancer, whereas an oxygen-rich, alkaline environment in the body could retain healthy cells.

In simple language, this means that acidic foods (such as meat, dairy products and sugar) can create an environment in the body that can lead to cancer, whereas alkaline foods (fruits, vegetables,

---

[2] The development of cancer occurs in three main stages, as follows:

Initiation – where normal genes become cancerous after chemicals are consumed and absorbed, then damaged DNA divides into new cells. This process can take only minutes to hours to occur.

Promotion – initiated cells continue to multiply if the conditions in the body allow and cluster together. This process takes years to decades to occur but can be reversible.

Progression – tumours develop from pre-cancerous cells, become more active and are eventually diagnosed as cancer. They can remain benign or infiltrate nearby tissue (metastasis), become aggressive and resistant to destruction.

wholegrains) can create an environment in the body that prevents the growth of cancer cells.

Dr Warburg's work was largely ignored within the medical community for a long time, until more recently as further research has come to light to support his claims. *The China Study* is one such example.

Breast and Prostate Cancer

The China Study determined that wealthy populations who consume the most meat and milk have higher rates of breast cancer. This indicates that environmental and dietary factors have more influence over disease than genetics. The three main contributors to breast cancer are the SAD, alcohol consumption and a sedentary lifestyle.

Studies on animals have also shown that if they are fed cow's milk and oestrogenic water, there are higher rates of breast cancer than if they are fed water or plant-based milks.

A study of 38 post-menopausal and overweight women who followed a plant-based diet and did moderate daily exercise for two weeks showed that their blood became less effective at growing breast cancer cells, and there was a higher rate of cells killing themselves off. *(Thomas Campbell, MD, Breast Cancer & Diet, 2020)*

A study undertaken in 2014 by the Bristol Nutrition Biomedical Research Unit found that men who eat more plant foods, with a high intake of fruits, vegetables and dietary fibre had a reduced risk of prostate cancer.

Despite the compelling evidence, there are no clinical trials of cancer patients eating a plant-based diet. Food as medicine has not been documented in scientific literature, and this is largely attributed to what was discussed earlier about nutritional paradigms and how these can determine where research funds are directed.

Angiogenesis

Angiogenesis is the process by which new blood vessels form and makes up part of the circulatory system. It's a vital function that needs to be balanced (not too many or too few blood vessels) so that all other systems associated with blood supply are healthy, too.

Inadequate blood vessel growth occurs in conditions such as heart failure, coronary heart disease and stroke. Excessive blood vessel growth occurs in conditions such as cancer, arthritis, Alzheimer's and diabetic blindness.

One way of treating cancer is through drugs that target angiogenesis – by limiting blood supply to the cancerous tumour. Many plant-based foods have been found to include antioxidants and anti-inflammatory properties that inhibit angiogenesis, such as fruits, vegetables, herbs, spices, tomatoes, berries, kale, and nuts. This presents the opportunity to include food, rather than just drugs, as a means of treatment for cancer patients.

Heart Disease

Cardiovascular disease is our top killer and is the cause of approximately 30% of deaths worldwide. There is a strong relationship between heart disease and the intake of animal protein, sugar, fat and total calories.

Dr William C Roberts, the editor in chief of the American Journal of Cardiology, states that cholesterol is the primary risk factor for atherosclerotic plaque build-up, specifically elevated LDL ('bad') cholesterol in the blood. To reduce LDL levels, three main things need to be reduced in the diet: trans-fat (found in processed foods, meat and dairy), saturated fat (found mainly in animal products and junk foods) and dietary cholesterol (found in animal-derived foods, especially eggs). *(Trumbo PR; Shimakawa T. Tolerable upper intake levels for trans-fat, saturated fat and cholesterol, Nutr Rev. 2011; 69(5):270-80)*

The common denominator in all of these is animal-based and processed junk foods.

A separate study carried out in the 1970s and published in the *Journal of Chronic Disease* in 1993 found that the following factors have a strong positive correlation to heart disease:

- Milk calcium
- Butterfat
- Saturated fat
- Calories from animal food
- Milk
- Milk protein
- Cholesterol
- Meat fat
- Meat protein.

A negative correlation to heart disease was found where diets contain more calories from vegetable foods, iron, starch and total carbohydrate compared with calories that came from animal foods.

International research and data has shown that populations with very low rates of heart disease (such as the Papua New Guinea islanders, the rural Chinese and the Okinawans in Japan) eat a primarily whole-food, plant-based diet with very little oil and refined sugar.

Populations such as the Inuit in the Arctic region and Masai in Africa have often been used as examples of why humans should follow a high-fat diet. The belief is that these people eat plenty of meat yet have a clean bill of health. This is not quite accurate.

In reality, the Masai don't eat nearly as much meat as we think, but they do have a diet high in milk. Autopsies have shown excessive atherosclerosis (hardening of the arteries) at similar levels to western men on the SAD, but it is believed that the Masai are protected from atherosclerosis by extreme amounts of physical exertion as part of their lifestyle which expand and enlargen their blood vessels. *(Spoerry A; Gray M; Jarashow D. Atherosclerosis in the Masai. Am J Epidemiol 95; 26-37, 1972)*

Autopsies on the Inuit show heart disease and deficient bone health as a result of diets high in protein, nitrogen and phosphorous and low in calcium.

An interesting trend was noted during World War II when the countries occupied by Germany had their livestock removed, such as Belgium, Holland, Norway and Denmark. There was a significant drop in deaths in these countries during that time, which then accelerated at the end of the war when they once more came to rely on livestock as a source of food.

The SAD, including foods such as oil, poultry, fish, meat, dairy, sugar and caffeine cause damage to endothelial cells (the lining of blood vessels). Studies have shown that a high intake of saturated fat causes the cells to become sticky and promotes plaque formation, which then blocks the arteries. *(Dow CA; Stauffer BL; Greiner JJ;*

et al, Influence of habitual high dietary fat intake on endothelium-dependent vasodilation)

Plant-based foods are packed with nitrates, which are then converted into nitric oxide in the body, and this prevents cellular stickiness, high blood pressure and plaque build-up.

People on the SAD also have a certain type of microbiota in their gut called carnitine and lecithin, which causes TMAO (a substance created in the liver and associated with the development of plaque in the arteries) and leads to a higher number of cardiac events. Those following a WFPB diet do not have these microbiota, so even if some meat is ingested, the body doesn't make TMAO.

Heart Health

Modern-day treatments for heart disease include stents, angioplasty and bypass surgery, all of which are risky, expensive and have an increased rate of failure over the long term. Even with all of these treatments, heart disease continues to be our number one killer in the western world, because while these advanced treatments can be incredible at saving lives, they are essentially an 'ambulance at the bottom of the cliff' approach.

There is some great evidence now that shows heart disease is reversible. Doctors specialising in plant-based nutrition such as Dean Ornish (Preventative Medicine Research Institute), Caldwell Esselstyn Jr (Cleveland Clinic) and the late Nathan Pritikin undertook a study to see what would happen when they put patients with advanced heart disease on a plant-based diet. The goal was to prevent progression of the disease, but incredibly, they found that the heart disease started to reverse. The patients stopped eating diets high in fat and ate plenty of vegetables, fruit and wholegrains. Plaque started to dissolve, and their arteries opened up. Leafy greens in particular were found to be phenomenal for the heath of endothelial cells.

This is an excellent example of the body having the innate ability to heal given the right tools and support. The body is desperate to be well!

Diabetes

Diabetes occurs when the pancreas is unable to produce enough insulin – an important hormone that regulates blood sugar and helps shuttle glucose from the blood stream into the cells. This causes raised glucose levels in the blood (known as hyperglycaemia), leading to damage to the body and failure of organs and tissues in the long term.

Type 1 Diabetes is an autoimmune condition that occurs when a damaged pancreas produces little or no insulin and is most commonly diagnosed in people under the age of 20.

Type 2 Diabetes is more common and has been called the *"black death of the twenty-first century."* It occurs when the body becomes resistant to insulin or when the pancreas doesn't produce enough insulin. This condition commonly affects overweight or obese adults. The term 'diabesity' has been coined as a result.

In 1935, Dr Rabinovitch, a physician from Montreal, carried out a study on a group of diabetic patients. Half were put on a low-carbohydrate diet, and the other half were put on a high-carbohydrate diet. After five years, 24% of patients in the high-carb group were able to come off insulin medication, whereas only 8% of the patients in the low-carb group could do the same. This study was instrumental in determining that a high-carb/high-fibre diet was good for diabetes. Further studies carried out in the 70s showed that patients were able to come off insulin after only three weeks on a high-fibre/high-carb, low-fat diet.

China is a very interesting case study in the area of diabetes. In 1991, 2.5% of the population had diabetes. Then came the availability of convenience and fast foods, and by 2000, this number had risen to 5.5%. Today, nearly half of the Chinese population is diabetic or pre-diabetic. *(Wang, L; Gao, P; Zhang, M; et al, JAMA Network, Prevalence and Ethnic Pattern of Diabetes and Pre-diabetes in China in 2013)*

High fat diets are strongly linked to diabetes. This is because fat blocks the muscle cells and prevents insulin from delivering glucose into the cells.

Insulin resistance is a process that starts many years before the diagnosis of diabetes. Behind the scenes, too many calories and too much fat in the diet creates a fatty liver, then the pancreas has to work extra hard to deal with the excess fat dumped by an overloaded liver into the bloodstream. A fatty liver and a damaged pancreas creates insulin resistance, raised blood sugar levels, and ultimately, leads to diabetes.

> *"Before diagnosis of Type 2 diabetes, there is a long, silent scream from the liver."*
>
> (Dr David Unwin)

On a WFPB diet where fats are kept relatively low, insulin is able to do its job more effectively. People following this diet have significantly less fat trapped in their muscle cells compared to people who eat meat. This means glucose can enter the cells more easily, resulting in more balanced blood sugar levels, better insulin sensitivity, and significantly better beta-cell function (cells that make insulin). *(Michael Greger, MD, FACLM, 2020)*

Studies on the effects of a WFPB diet on the treatment of diabetes are telling. One study carried out in 2005 by Dr Neal Barnard took diabetic patients with Type 2 diabetes and placed them on a vegan diet, with minimal oil consumption and low glycaemic index (GI) foods. Blood sugar levels rapidly decreased, even more so than for people on oral diabetic medications. Cholesterol and blood pressure improved, and weight loss happened easily. These patients were tracked for an additional year and managed to maintain their results, while reducing or completely eliminating their diabetic medication.

When diabetic patients visit their GP, they are being told to stop eating fruit because of the high sugar content. Can you believe it? Stop eating the food that has the absolute best power to heal the body? Yes, this is what we're dealing with when it comes to conventional medicine treating chronic disease and shows how far removed from common sense we have become. All our diabetic clients eat fruit, and their bodies start to heal. Natural sugars from fruit are not the problem when it comes to diabetes. Fatty diets are the problem.

Epigenetics

Research by Dr Dean Ornish has shown that genetics play a far less significant role in chronic disease than once thought. Rather, genes are the 'loaded gun', and lifestyle choices are the 'trigger.' In other words, just because you may have a predisposition towards a certain disease because one of your parents developed that disease, your lifestyle choices actually determine whether you will develop that disease up to 95% of the time. Dr Ornish's research has shown that gene expression can change significantly after just three months of comprehensive lifestyle and diet changes, particularly the genes that cause oxidative stress and inflammation.

Positive lifestyle changes can lengthen telomeres (the ends of chromosomes that control our lifespan). This is a fascinating field of research because it essentially shows that ageing can be reversed at a cellular level.

What this tells us is that the body can heal itself relatively rapidly when it's given the correct support via food.

Environmental Impacts

While the environmental impacts of meat production are not my area of expertise or the focus of this book, it is a massive problem and deserves mention here. These days there is a high level of awareness about adverse environmental effects from the production of meat, but it's still happening at an alarming rate due to hunger for profit and society's dreadful eating habits.

Bruce Monger, PhD is a teacher of ocean remote sensing at Cornell University and points to farming practices as the primary cause of water pollution because too many nutrients such as phosphorous and nitrogen are leached into the water and act like fertiliser. This then leads to excessive algae growth, which blocks sunlight, reduces oxygen and creates an uninhabitable environment for marine life. New Zealand, with its high use of fertilisers, has a 'dead zone' problem in its oceans, where oxygen levels plummet so low that marine life can't survive.

The United Nations has called for a global reduction in meat and dairy consumption because the methane produced from livestock digestion, nitrous oxide from increased use of fertilisers and carbon dioxide from clearing and burning forests to grow food for livestock contribute to over half of greenhouse gas emissions every year. There is also increasing concern about the outlook for growing crops amid climate change and the ability to feed the world's population.

Overfishing is also a significant problem. Large companies with little concern for conservation are depleting fish stocks and in the process are creating problems with bycatch, where unwanted sea life is being captured while trawling for a different species. This creates needless loss of billions of fish which is a serious problem for countries who rely on fish as a staple in their diet. Longline fishing – where baited hooks are over 100km long – is also detrimental to birds and sharks.

All of these practices are a result of the demand for meat, and they are basically destroying our ecosystem, which then affects things like clean water supply and leads to deforestation and lack of protection from natural disasters.

GMOs (Genetically Modified Organisms) create problems because the most common GMO plants – such as maize and soybeans – are becoming resistant to herbicides and insecticides, which means farmers spray them more often to ensure maximum yield from their crops. Glyphosate is a problematic herbicide which has been categorised as a probable carcinogen for humans and a contributor to endocrine disruption and Parkinsons. It also disrupts the nutrient balance in plants. Interestingly, many of the same companies who are involved in developing GMO plants are also developing the sprays, which raises questions around ethical behaviour.

Water

Did you know it takes one hundred times more water to produce a pound of animal protein than it does to produce a pound of grain protein? The Water Footprint Network (waterfootprint.org) is an informative website where you can find information on the impact your lifestyle and dietary choices have on the world's freshwater supply.

Plastics and Packaging

Many of the materials used for plastic packaging for our food are non-recyclable and can end up where they shouldn't be, such as the ocean. Many countries are now suffering the fall-out from devastating water pollution, which of course has a roll-on effect to sea life.

An added benefit when you follow a plant-based diet is that the amount of plastic packaging you use decreases significantly because you are no longer purchasing as many processed foods. If you buy fresh produce and things like grains or nuts and seeds in bulk, your trips to the trash bin become few and far between.

Below are some ways you can create a low-waste, plant-based home, simply through changing some daily habits:

- Take your own grocery bags to the supermarket. Thankfully in NZ and several other countries, plastic bags are no longer used to pack groceries at the supermarket. They still sell them though! Aim to reduce the number of plastic bags you use at home.

- Take cloth bags for dry goods, or jars for liquid items to places that sell grocery items in bulk.
- Use designated recycling bins – make use of the designated bins provided by your local council to prevent unnecessary rubbish going to landfill.
- Swap disposable for re-useable – use cloth kitchen towels and napkins instead of the paper variety. Resist using plastic lunch bags and invest in containers or silicon storage bags instead. Glass storage containers are ideal for snacks and leftovers at home.
- Take a packed lunch – convenience foods and takeaways generally use plastic packaging, so use a lunch box with a set of re-useable utensils and take lunch from home. Cheaper, healthier and environmentally friendly!
- Use a multi-purpose drink bottle for beverages to avoid single-use coffee-cups and plastic bottles.
- Avoid plastic straws because they block our waterways and damage sea life. Paper and biodegradable straws still create unnecessary waste. Use stainless steel or bamboo straws instead.

If your lingering thoughts after reading this chapter are, *"How depressing,"* I hear you. The human race really does seem to be intent on screwing things up, doesn't it? With how we are treating ourselves and our environment, the future doesn't look bright at all. It's a huge area of concern and it feels insurmountable.

However, massive global change happens when individuals decide to make a stand and do things differently. Yes, it takes time, but we must start somewhere. Your decision to take responsibility for your health and our environment won't change the world, but it will change *your* world and have positive impacts on the people around you.

And that's an excellent place to start.

Digging up the Dirt

Close your eyes and visualise yourself in 10 or 20 years' time. If you continue with your current lifestyle and eating habits, what is your physical, mental and emotional health like? Now do the same again, but imagine you have a healthy, nutritious diet. What is your life like in this scenario?

_____

_____

_____

_____

_____

_____

_____

_____

_____

_____

_____

CHAPTER FOUR
Nourishing Nutrition

Nutrition is a very broad topic and if you go to your public library or local bookstore, you can spend endless hours thumbing through rows of books on the subject. That's the best approach if you want to end up thoroughly overwhelmed and confused – I've been there, done that and can speak from experience!

When I was really sick and decided to focus on my diet as a means of recovery, I didn't have the energy or desire to plough through stacks of books which, a lot of the time, contradicted one another. I needed something I could trust to be reliable, accurate, and most of all, logical. Eating tons of fat every day on the Keto diet didn't sound logical. Significantly reducing carbohydrate intake didn't sound logical. Eating only between certain hours of the day didn't sound logical. Cutting out fruit sounded outright ludicrous.

Eating plenty of fresh, natural, nutrient-dense foods provided by nature? Now that sounded like something I could get on board with. But more importantly, it just felt right. I couldn't argue with evidence showing me that eating things like fruits, vegetables and wholegrains grown from the earth was going to be good for me. If it's a down-to-earth approach, I'm probably going to like it!

Doctor *Google* provides many different definitions of nutrition, but most of them reflect the study of nutrients in isolation. Wait a minute. Does this sound familiar? Do you remember our discussion about the 'reductionist' viewpoint in Chapter Two, where body parts and disease are treated in isolation, too? There's definitely a trend going on here!

A traditional explanation of nutrition goes like this:

> *"Nutrition is the biochemical and physiological process by which an organism uses food to support its life. It includes ingestion, absorption, assimilation, biosynthesis, catabolism and excretion."*
>
> (Wikipedia)

Now contrast this with Dr T Colin Campbell's definitions:

> *"Nutrition is the biologically (w)holistic process by which elements of food and water are used by the body to optimise health."*
>
> (Dr T Colin Campbell)

and

Nourishing Nutrition

> *"Nutrition is the highly integrated reactions and events of countless food chemicals working together, as in a symphony."*
>
> (Dr T Colin Campbell)

Can you see the difference?

Dr Campbell's definitions more accurately reflect the relationship between nutrition and health, a relationship that is not fully explored or given enough gravity by conventional medicine.

We have already discussed the varied reasons why people eat the way they do. One of them is confusion, or a basic lack of understanding about what good nutrition actually means. Without this basic understanding, we are immediately on the back-foot in knowing how to nourish our bodies correctly, and we certainly won't be questioning whether our current habits are working for or against us.

We must educate ourselves on good nutrition to provide the foundations from which our bodies and minds can start to flourish, and also to be able to pass our knowledge on to future generations – who are being misled by rich and powerful industries in the forms of snazzy TV commercials about their 'healthy' and 'nutritious' food.

In this chapter, we are going to explore the different types of nutrients, the comparison in nutrients between animal-based diets and plant-based diets, how to interpret food labels, and where to source essential nutrients.

A nutrient is a compound in food that can't be made by the body and therefore must be consumed and assists in creating and restoring health. There are seven types of nutrients:

1. Protein
2. Carbohydrates
3. Fats (Macronutrients)
4. Vitamins and Minerals (Micronutrients)
5. Phytonutrients
6. Fibre
7. Water.

It is believed that there are still several nutrients yet to be identified.

Protein

Protein is an essential nutrient for the body and is considered the 'building block' of tissues, organs and multiple bodily functions. It is made up of a chain of 20 amino acids linked together, nine of which the human body can't make itself so needs to obtain from food. Its main function is the formation of enzymes (molecules in the body that control metabolism).

Protein has been the 'favourite child' of all the nutrients in the study of nutrition throughout history. Western society seems to have an obsession with protein; the fear of not getting enough, a belief that more is better, and we tend to associate strength, size and ability with more protein. In fact, the word protein derives from the Greek word *"proteios"*, which translates as *"prime importance"*.

Animal foods have generally been regarded as high-quality proteins because it is believed they are used more efficiently by the body and have a higher biological value (BV) than plant-based proteins. However, research through *The China Study* showed that proteins with a higher BV can result in detrimental effects on the body, including cancer growth rates, stimulation of growth factors and body growth rates, and are a trigger for early menstruation and breast cancer in females.

It was found that even though high-quality animal protein promotes efficient growth, plant-based proteins cause less *unwanted* growth and fulfil our dietary needs perfectly, despite not matching the human amino acid profile. *(T Colin Campbell, 2020)*

The first question that most people get asked when they transition to a WFPB diet is, *"But, where will you get your protein?"*

Given the recommended dietary allowance of protein for humans is 8-10% of calories, which is easily achieved by eating a variety of plant-based foods, this is a non-issue for vegans or followers of the plant-based lifestyle.

Think about the last time you heard about anyone with a protein deficiency. I bet you never have! Think about animals who thrive on plants, such as gorillas, zebras and elephants. Does anyone worry about where they get their protein from? Do these animals look like they are weak and malnourished? Of course not! They are perfectly strong and healthy, and they get all the protein they need from plants.

Eating an excess of animal protein is actually detrimental to our health because it creates extra stress on the kidneys, liver and bones. *(Delimaris, I, Adverse effects associated with protein intake above the recommended dietary allowance for adults, ISRN Nutr. 2013)*

Contrary to popular belief, protein does not create muscle mass. The amount of muscle we have is determined by genetics, hormones and the frequency with which muscle is loaded (i.e. weightlifting).

As more comes to light about the benefit of a WFPB diet, even high performing and endurance athletes are thriving on this diet and experiencing superior performance. The world's strongest man, Patrik Baboumian is a vegan, which goes against everything we have been taught about animal protein being required for superior strength.

As long as you are eating plenty of plant-based foods, you don't need to worry about protein!

Protein-rich plant-based foods include tofu, tempeh, edamame, lentils, chickpeas, peanuts, almonds, spirulina, quinoa, chia seeds, hemp seeds, beans with rice, potatoes and leafy green vegetables.

Carbohydrates

The digestive system converts carbohydrates into simple sugars like glucose (blood sugar) and they become the body's main energy source. There are three main types of carbohydrates: sugar, starch and fibre, and they can be defined as simple or complex, depending on their chemical structure.

Simple carbs provide a source of quick energy, and complex carbs are broken down more slowly and provide longer lasting energy. Common sources include fruit, vegetables, nuts, grains, seeds and legumes.

Refined carbohydrates are created through processes that reduce or remove fibre, antioxidants, vitamins, minerals and phytochemicals. These processes can also add fat (trans and saturated) and sugar. Too many refined carbohydrates in the diet can cause insulin problems, and combined with fat, can lead to weight gain. Common sources include white grains and flours, sugars, syrups, candy and pastries.

The belief that 'carbs are bad' or 'carbs will make you fat' is misguided and factually incorrect. In reality, an ideal WFPB lifestyle includes 80% of energy from carbs! Low-carb diets can be damaging because they limit the consumption of plants. This leads to excessive consumption of protein and fat, resulting in dietary imbalances associated with high rates of chronic disease.

A high complex carb, high vegetable diet typically leads to low body mass, whereas high animal protein diets are associated with higher body mass. What this tells us is that carbohydrates are not causing chronic disease; excess fat and processed foods are.

Fibre

Fibre is a type of carbohydrate found only in plants which helps to regulate the body's use of sugars and reduce hunger. The body can't digest fibre because it can't be broken down into sugar molecules.

There are two types of fibre. Soluble fibre absorbs water and forms a gel-like texture which is digested by gut bacteria and turned into usable energy. Insoluble fibre doesn't absorb water, passes through the body without changing much and adds bulk to stools. The majority of fibre in our diets is insoluble.

The health effects of fibre are vast, which makes it a super important part of our diet. Benefits include:

- Slowing down how quickly food passes through the stomach.

- Making you feel full for longer (for example, oranges which have fibre, compared with orange juice which has none).
- Lowering cholesterol levels.
- Helping produce short-chain fatty acids which create a healthy gut environment.
- Reducing inflammation in the gut.
- Improving bowel health and reducing the onset of inflammatory bowel diseases, cardiovascular disease and diabetes.

A WFPB diet offers significantly more fibre per day compared with the SAD. I I don't think I need to tell you what this means when it comes to strained versus smooth bowel movements!

Good sources of fibre include raw strawberries, raw almonds, oats, whole flaxseeds, cooked navy beans, kidney beans, pinto beans, chickpeas and lentils, barley flour, dry roasted nuts and pumpkin seeds and raw avocados.

Grains

Grains are seeds harvested for human or animal consumption. A wholegrain is a grain that contains the endosperm, germ and bran. In contrast, refined grains are grains that have been significantly modified from their natural composition, involving a process that mechanically removes the germ and bran and their associated nutrients. Refined grains lose up to 80% of their nutrients during this process and many are not supplemented with vitamins and minerals, so are much less nutrient-dense than wholegrains.

Refined grains include macaroni, spaghetti, grits, pretzels, puffed rice/wheat, corn flakes, crisped rice, degermed cornmeal, white bread and white rice.

Whole grains include corn, quinoa, spelt, wheat, oat, barley (not pearl), brown rice, wild rice, millet and buckwheat.

From a health perspective, it's always best to choose wholegrains and avoid refined grains as much as possible.

A Note on Gluten

Gluten has become a big problem in recent years because the type of wheat we eat now is very different to what our grandparents ate. Today's wheat is the product of cross-breeding and genetic manipulation to create higher-yielding, lower cost crops. It's also heavily bleached and processed and essential nutrients have been removed. Combine this with the prevalence of gut issues in the general population and we end up with significant problems. I take all my clients off gluten, and this is particularly important for those with inflammatory gut or bowel problems, autoimmune dysfunction or problematic skin.

Fats

Fats play an important role in the body. Primarily, their role is to store energy, protect the organs, support cell growth, control cholesterol and blood pressure, and help the body absorb essential nutrients.

On the SAD, fats make up approximately 30-50% of the diet, mostly in the form of animal-based foods and fats/oils. On a WFPB diet, fats make up just 10-12% of the diet. This goes a long way to explaining why generally, one's waistline tends to be smaller on a plant-based diet.

Fatty acids on a plant-based diet are mainly unsaturated fatty acids, whereas fatty acids from animal-based foods are mainly saturated.

You have most likely heard of omega 3 and omega 6 fats. Both are essential, but omega 3 are anti-inflammatory, while omega 6 are pro-inflammatory. Inflammation created by omega 6 is not completely detrimental; it's actually an important part of healing and correct immune function. However, the correct balance of omega 6 to omega 3 is essential to promote inflammation that assists in healing, whereas imbalances can lead to chronic and problematic inflammation.

Ideally, the ratio of omega 6 to omega 3 in the diet should be 1:1. A WFPB lifestyle provides a ratio of 1:1 to 3:1. The SAD provides a ratio of 20:1 to 50:1. Can you believe it? No wonder people who follow the SAD are so sick!

Many people like to obtain omega 3 and 6 in the form of supplements, but this approach overlooks the underlying issues that cause imbalances to begin with and doesn't address them. Certain lifestyle factors can adversely affect the absorption of omega 3, such as the use of prescription medication, alcohol consumption, vitamin/mineral deficiencies, a compromised immune system and a high-fat diet.

Obtaining essential fatty acids from food is always the best approach. Excellent plant-based sources of omega 3 include avocados, ground flaxseed, chia seeds, hemp seeds, walnuts, brussels sprouts and leafy greens.

Good sources of plant-based omega 6 include tofu, peanut butter, avocados, walnuts, hemp seeds and soybeans.

Trans-fats are very detrimental to our health and raise our LDL cholesterol ('bad' cholesterol) and lowers our HDL cholesterol ('good' cholesterol). Mostly, trans-fats occur when unsaturated fats are hydrogenated (have hydrogen atoms added to them). Manipulating the amount of hydrogen in food changes the food's characteristics and can cause detrimental health effects. Cooking oils are often hydrogenated to make them more suitable for frying food and to give them a longer shelf life, but this process can cause cells in the body to calcify, create inflammation in the arteries and is also linked to other chronic disease.

Common foods with trans-fats include pastries, crackers, popcorn, frozen pizza, margarine, biscuits, icing and fried food.

Macronutrients in Animal vs Plant Foods

The nutritional makeup of foods is a broad and complex topic, but much of the research into the WFPB diet points to the superiority of plant foods over animal-based foods.

Here are some interesting facts to know:

- Plant foods are abundant in carbohydrates.
- Protein is contained in all whole foods.
- Only plants contain beta-carotene (a pigment that converts into Vitamin A).
- Vitamin C, Vitamin E, folate, iron, magnesium and calcium are much higher in plants than in animal foods.
- Nuts and seeds are high in fat and protein but are healthier than animal-based protein.
- Processed plant foods are deficient in protein.
- Processed plant foods are abundant in carbohydrates, but

these come from white flour or sugar and are deficient in fibre.
- There is fat in whole plants but to a lesser extent than in refined plant foods or animal foods.
- Plants contain no cholesterol.[3]

In summary, a WFPB (high-carbohydrate) diet will lead to good health and a lower risk for chronic illness. A diet high in animal foods and processed plant foods will lead to chronic disease and a painful trip down Medication Alley with your doctor.

Much to the frustration of leaders in the plant-based nutrition research field, long-standing beliefs around nutrition means that research in this area continues to be biased against a WFPB diet and many people remain unaware that the answer to their health issues lies within this way of eating. Hopefully as the findings from doctors and scientists who continue to research this way of eating becomes more widespread, and if society can shift towards a more 'wholistic' view of nutrition, bias and confusion will become a thing of the past.

Interpreting Food Labels

In 2002, a law was introduced in New Zealand where all foods had to include a nutrition label. A back-of-pack nutritional information panel (NIP) must display the content of energy (calories or kilojoules), fat, saturated fat, protein, carbohydrate, sugar and sodium per serving and per 100g of food. Generally, this practice isn't particularly effective, mainly because many consumers have a very limited understanding on how to interpret the labels, and simply ignore them altogether.

---

[3] *(Source: T Colin Campbell, 2020).*

Nourishing Nutrition

Part of educating yourself about good nutrition is learning how to interpret one of these labels. Once you know how, it's quite easy and it can help you figure out whether you should put a certain food item in your trolley, or back on the supermarket shelf.

The table below is taken from the back of a standard chocolate bar, followed by instructions on how to interpret it.

NUTRITION INFORMATION
SERVINGS PER PACKAGE: 1
SERVING SIZE: 50g

Average Quantities	Per Serving	%DI Per Serve*	Per 100g
ENERGY	1030kJ	12%	2020kJ
PROTEIN	4.4g	9%	8.7g
FAT – Total	12.2g	17%	24.0g
– Saturated	4.5g	19%	8.8g
CARBOHYDRATE	28.6g	9%	56.5g
– Sugars	25.6g	28%	50.6g
SODIUM	119mg	5%	236mg

The first thing to look at is how many servings there are in the packet, and in this case, there is one, so the nutrition information provided relates to the whole bar of chocolate.

Then, we work out how many calories are in the chocolate bar by dividing the number of kilojoules by 4.2 (there are 4.2 kilojoules in one calorie).

1030 / 4.2 = 246 calories (rounded up)

Next, we look at how the number of calories is distributed between fat, carbohydrate and protein. All numbers are rounded up to the nearest whole number.

Fat
Each gram of fat has 9 calories, so 12.2g of fat x 9 calories = **110 calories**

Carbohydrate
Each gram of carbohydrate has 4 calories, so 28.6g of carbohydrate x 4 calories = **115 calories**

Protein
Each gram of protein has 4 calories, so 4.4g of protein x 4 calories = **18 calories**

Now, we work out the percentages of fat, carbohydrate and protein in the chocolate bar. All numbers are rounded up to the nearest whole number.

Fat
110 calories as a percentage of 246 (total calories) = 45%

Carbohydrate
115 calories as a percentage of 246 (total calories) = 47%

Protein
18 calories as a percentage of 246 (total calories) = 8%

So, as you can see, the chocolate bar contains 45% fat, which means *almost half of the bar is pure fat!* Do you still want to eat it after knowing that?

As you've already discovered, the food and beverage industry doesn't exactly adhere to high morals and standards in their tactics when selling to consumers, and even though lawfully they must provide nutritional information, by and large it won't adversely affect them because nobody knows what on earth the labels mean. We know these large industries don't give a hoot about what their products are doing to our health, and the only way we can protect ourselves is to become educated and be more discerning about what we buy.

You can practice interpreting labels with foods off the supermarket shelf, or even by going into your pantry and looking at what's already there. I guarantee you will start to reassess some of the common, every-day foods you are buying that promise 'natural' and 'healthy' ingredients on the front of the box. The harsh reality is that you are most likely consuming a whole lot of fat and other nasty ingredients which will make you sick.

Where to Get Essential Nutrients

A WFPB lifestyle will provide you with almost every nutrient you need. Vitamin supplements are all the rage these days, but this is often because trendy diets (such as Atkins or Keto) promote illness which then require followers of these diets to take supplements to restore health. Many of the people fronting these types of trend diets have a lucrative side-business of selling supplements – talk about unethical!

Vitamin supplements should not be viewed as a cure-all. They may go some way to preventing deficiencies in the short-term, but there is little evidence to suggest they create long-term health benefits.

With this in mind, there are a few key areas to consider when following a WFPB diet, outlined below:

Vitamin B12

Vitamin B12 is required to form red blood cells and DNA, and plays a key role in a healthy brain and nervous system. It's a myth that people who don't eat meat are at the greatest risk for a Vitamin B12 deficiency. In truth, even heavy consumers of meat can be deficient. Just because blood tests may show you have adequate supplies of Vitamin B12, it doesn't mean it is able to be correctly utilised by the brain or central nervous system. In our coaching practice, we recommend everyone take a B12 supplement because it is antiviral, supports liver function, the brain and central nervous system.

Plant foods containing good sources of B12: nutritional yeast, fortified cereals and milks, mushrooms, algae, spinach, beetroot, potatoes and alfalfa.

Iron

Ensure you are eating plenty of iron rich foods such as grains, dark leafy vegetables, legumes, nuts and seeds. It's best to pair these foods with foods rich in Vitamin C for better absorption. Dairy products are actually one of the biggest risk factors contributing to iron deficiency because they are very low in iron and replace the calories from healthier foods. Dairy also interferes with iron absorption and can cause micro-haemorrhage in the gut, leading to iron loss. *(Jackie Busse, MD, 2020)*

Plant foods containing good sources of iron: lentils, chickpeas, beans, tofu, cashew nuts, chia seeds, ground linseed, hemp seeds, pumpkin seeds, kale, dried apricots, dried figs, raisins, quinoa and fortified breakfast cereal.

Calcium

There is no solid evidence linking calcium to bone health. In fact, data shows that the countries with the highest calcium intake have the highest rate of osteoporosis. *(Mahdi, A; Brown, R; Razzaque, M. Osteoporosis in Populations with High Calcium Intake, Indian Journal of Clinical Biochemistry, 2015)*

Factors important for bone health include weight-bearing exercise, adequate Vitamin D (sunshine), a low sodium diet, avoiding excess dietary protein (especially animal protein), and maintaining an alkaline diet rich in fruits and vegetables. *(Jackie Busse, 2020)*

Plant foods containing good sources of calcium: bok choy, kale, mustard greens, turnip greens, watercress, broccoli, chickpeas, tofu, beans, nuts and seeds, fortified plant milks and juices.

Vitamin D

This is actually a hormone, not a vitamin. It is unrelated to diet and is only found in dairy products because it is added artificially. Humans make Vitamin D from sunshine, and this is the best way to get it. We need 15-20 minutes of midday sun exposure without sunblock each day, where 50-70% of the skin is exposed. People who live in areas a long way from the equator who cannot access adequate sunlight are recommended to take a Vitamin D supplement. Also keep in mind that darker skin will require additional time in the sun.

If you notice any adverse changes in your health after beginning a WFPB lifestyle, I recommend speaking to your healthcare professional. It is also a good idea to get regular blood tests, especially for iron, ferritin and B12. You may wish to take a good quality multi-vitamin supplement for the first few months while you learn more about your new way of eating and become familiar with healthy eating patterns. If you do take supplements, make sure to check the appropriate dosage and if unsure, speak to your pharmacist.

Phytonutrients

Phytonutrients are natural compounds found in plant foods such as fruits, vegetables, legumes and wholegrains. They provide antioxidants, have anti-inflammatory properties and can enhance immunity and DNA repair from exposure to toxins and carcinogens. Eating at least five portions of fruits and vegetables each day will ensure a good intake of phytonutrients.

Water

We all know how important water is for human survival, and adults should be drinking at least 2.5 litres of water per day, or even more during hot temperatures or for someone with an active lifestyle. This will ensure adequate hydration so that all functions of the body can perform optimally. A good test for hydration is to check the colour of your urine – it should run clear.

In my opinion, the evidence for following a WFPB diet is very compelling, not only because I've done the research, but more importantly, I see the evidence in myself every single day. Never before have I felt so energetic, alive and well, and everyone I work with who adopts this lifestyle says the same thing for themselves.

As with anything new though, it's natural to have some scepticism. Perhaps your best friend follows a high-fat diet and raves about it and thinks you're mad if you want to eat all those carbs. From my personal experience in my coaching practice, many of my clients have tried high-fat diets and have ended up with bigger problems than they started with.

This is a good example of where it's really important to take a step back, think logically and adopt some common sense. Does it sound sensible to avoid fruit and eat tons of fat in the form of butter and bacon? Was butter and bacon put on this earth to nourish human beings and help them thrive? Does their dull colour represent freshness and vibrancy? Does the fact that the digestive system will struggle to break down those fatty foods and make you constipated sound healthy?

Common sense tells us that no, it doesn't. And don't get me started on the bulletproof coffee trend of putting pure butter into your coffee…

Perhaps you love meat and worry about going hungry without it. I can assure you that once you start eating whole, fresh, nutrient-dense foods, your body will get everything it needs, and hunger won't even be an issue. You'll also notice your tastebuds starting to change quite quickly, and before you know it, a whole week will go by, and you haven't even thought about meat! And if you do feel like a piece from time to time, there's nothing stopping you – this is the 'wriggle' room I referred to earlier.

If you think it all sounds too hard to change because of your conditioning, or tastebuds, or preferences, or because your family and friends will scoff at you, let me tell you what's even harder.

Spending a lifetime plodding through weeks, months and years feeling like life is passing you by and watching your dreams fade and die. Coming to the end of your life and regretting all the things you didn't or couldn't do because you didn't have the energy, or motivation, or belief. Experiencing a health crisis so devastating that it cuts your life short. A deep knowing that you had more in you, and you wasted it.

Those things are hard.

When you look at it that way, making adjustments to how you eat doesn't sound so difficult after all, does it?

And trust me when I say, it's the one thing that will transform your world and enable you to live the life you dream of.

Digging up the Dirt

Are your current dietary habits giving you adequate nutrition? Which areas are lacking and what changes do you need to make?

CHAPTER FIVE
Potent Plants

We've talked about the incredible ability of the WFPB diet to drastically reduce rates of chronic illness such as heart disease, cancer and diabetes, but there's so much more to know when it comes to all the positive things this way of life brings.

In my coaching practice, I see the whole spectrum of health issues and I never tire of seeing the incredible results that unfold when people start eating fresh, nutrient-dense, whole foods. When they first come to see me, many of my clients haven't given much thought to following a plant-based diet because they either don't understand what it is, or they are under the impression that they will have to survive on lentils and lettuce leaves.

There are so many things to love about this way of life, but one that really stands out for me is the pure freedom you can experience by eating this way. There's the misconception that the WFPB diet is restrictive and dull, but actually the opposite is true.

Never have I experienced so much freedom in my life.

Not once while following this lifestyle have I ever weighed or measured my food, or counted calories, or obsessed about carbs vs protein vs fat. I know that as long as there is a good variety of fresh and brightly coloured foods on my plate at each meal, I am getting all the goodness I need, and in the right quantities. As long as I tune in and pay attention to what my body is telling me, my portion sizes will be spot on.

Often when I show my clients the meal plans on my coaching programme, there is an audible sigh of relief once they realise calorie counting and measuring portion sizes are not required. Our bodies have an innate ability to know how much to eat and when to stop, but our modern habit of living on junk foods loaded with artificial ingredients has destroyed that ability. Our addiction to ridiculous quantities of sugar, fat and salt have completely annihilated our brain's capacity to regulate and control genuine hunger, so we end up stuffing ourselves silly.

There is an incredible bounty of food available to us when we divert our eyes from all the processed and packaged rubbish. The next time you go to the supermarket, really look at the abundance of fresh fruits and vegetables on display. Row after row after row! One of the best things about starting to eat fresh foods is that as your taste buds quickly change, you will start to crave these foods more and more.

I always make an allowance for my clients to have a cheat meal each week where they can indulge in anything they like, but after a few weeks on the programme, they no longer enjoy them because they realise how lousy they feel afterwards. It's a great way to teach them that their bodies are communicating with them all the time, and that their various niggly symptoms that return after a cheat meal are a sign that something's not right.

Since following this way of life, I have not once worried about eating 'good' foods or 'bad' foods. I know that as long as I am eating fresh, nutrient-dense foods 85-90% of the time, I can enjoy some delicious treats the rest of the time and my health or waistline won't suffer.

Not only this, but I also have the freedom in knowing that my body is going to cooperate with everything I need and want to do. I can do whatever exercise I choose, I can get out of the bed in the morning pain-free, I can trust my mind to be focused and stable, I can rely on great sleep most of the time, I am able to moderate my stress levels well... And the list goes on.

I feel better at 44 years old than I ever have in my life.

I know there are no guarantees when it comes to health, but I feel confident in my choices because my body is communicating to me every day that it is well.

> "The body is always talking to you. What do you do when you get a message from your body, such as a little ache or pain? Usually, you run to the medicine cabinet and take a pill. In effect, you say to the body, 'Shut up! I don't want to hear you. Don't talk to me!'"
>
> (Louise Hay)

Most people are very good at telling their bodies to shut up, rather than really tuning in and listening to what they are saying. The beauty of the WFPB diet is that you learn to listen to what your body is trying to communicate with you. Then, once you are clear with what's wrong, you can take the required action to address it.

I would need to write another entire book to cover all the benefits of a plant-based diet as it relates to improving one's wellbeing (and I might one day!) but for now let's take a deeper look at just a few of the key ways in which a WFPB diet has a positive impact on various aspects of health.

Allergies

As a self-confessed 'allergic person' who has struggled with eczema, asthma and hay fever for most of my life, I can tell you from first-hand experience that a WFPB diet is second-to-none for getting on top of these issues. Gone are the days when I need to take my Ventolin inhaler everywhere I go or deal with raw, cracked and itchy skin. By default, a WFPB diet removes common allergens such as dairy products (milk, cheese, yoghurt), and eggs. I know without a doubt when a food with dairy products has snuck in, because my airways immediately close and I am grasping for my inhaler.

I also take all my clients off gluten, which is another problematic food for allergies. The beauty of the WFPB diet is that it is still rich in grains, and there are plenty of great gluten-free varieties available these days.

The SAD weakens the immune system and causes gut problems, which allows for allergies to creep in. A diet high in fruits, vegetables and wholegrains heals the gut, lowers inflammation in the body and strengthens the immune system, drastically reducing the chance of allergies. In fact, a diet high in fruits, vegetables and wholegrains lowers the probability of being asthmatic by 66%. *(Tabak C; Wigg AH. The International Study on Allergy and Asthma in Childhood, Utrecht University. 1991, ongoing study)*

Autoimmune Dysfunction

When underlying viral activity in the body is treated (specifically the Epstein-Barr Virus), problematic symptoms associated with autoimmune dysfunction start to vanish. Part of a holistic treatment protocol for viral activity is to remove sources of fuel which cause viral activity to thrive – such as dairy products, gluten and eggs. Most people with autoimmune conditions go to their doctor and are told their body is attacking itself, or that nothing can be done, and they will need to rely on medication for life. This is an unhelpful approach to say the least.

I have treated numerous clients who suffer from autoimmune dysfunction with an anti-inflammatory, anti-viral, WFPB diet, and see them watch in disbelief as their troublesome symptoms start to disappear – and quite quickly, too.

Brain Health

Strokes and Alzheimer's are the two most serious brain diseases. Most strokes are caused by a clogged artery blocking blood flow to the brain. There are numerous studies now to show that high fibre, potassium, citrus and antioxidant intake reduces the risk of stroke, all of which occur naturally in the WFPB diet.

Currently there is no cure for Alzheimer's disease and little progress is being made within conventional medicine to understanding it. On a positive note, some doctors and scientists are now saying that while there is no cure, it can be prevented through diet and lifestyle changes, specifically by replacing meat and dairy products with vegetables, legumes and wholegrains as primary staples of the diet. *(Barnard, ND; Bush, AI; Ceccarelli, A; et al. Dietary and Lifestyle Guidelines for the prevention of Alzheimer's disease, Neurobiol Aging. 2014; 35 Suppl 2:S74-8)*

Energy Levels

The body depends on carbohydrates as its primary source of fuel, and that's why low-carb diets typically don't work over the long term. The body can't perform optimally when it's running short on glucose from carbs and will end up releasing excess stress hormones such as adrenaline to enable to the body to function, leading to a whole host of problems. The ideal ratio of carbs in a WFPB diet is a whopping 80%, made up of mostly fruits, vegetables and wholegrains. The fibre, complex carbs and water content in these foods provide a slow release of glucose, which promotes stable energy levels throughout the day.

Gut and Digestive Health

A healthy gut with healthy stomach acids breaks down and digests food and absorbs nutrients correctly. If the gut is in a mess, symptoms like constipation, diarrhoea, bloating, cramps and pain can be the result. The fresh, nutrient-dense foods on a WFPB diet are packed with probiotics (particularly fresh fruits and vegetables) that flood the gut with beneficial bacteria and promote healthy acids. The SAD on the other hand strips away essential stomach acids and promotes 'bad' gut bacteria, which has flow-on effects to many other functions in the body.

Hormonal Balance

Many factors can cause hormonal imbalances in the body, including illnesses such as thyroiditis and diabetes, cancer treatments, medications, chemicals, stress, inflammatory foods and poor sleep. Farming-related practices, such as feeding animals antibiotics and keeping cows pregnant to maximise dairy output create high levels of oestrogen which adversely affect hormones for both men and women. Plant-based foods such as cruciferous vegetables, essential fatty acids, healthy fats, turmeric and ginger, adaptogens (herbs promoting hormonal health), fibre, berries and cinnamon help balance hormones by detoxifying oestrogen from the body.

Liver Health

In my coaching programme, I put a lot of emphasis on healing the liver because it is such a crucial organ that is responsible for over 2,000 functions in the body. Most people have a sick liver due to poor lifestyle choices – fatty foods, caffeine, sugar and alcohol – and inflammation or viral infection that often resides there. The most serious liver conditions, such as liver failure, liver cancer and cirrhosis are generally caused by inflammation, so it makes perfect sense that a diet full of anti-inflammatory foods such as those on the WFPB diet is going to prevent and in some cases, reverse liver problems. Oats and cranberries are particularly protective foods for the liver.

Menopause Symptoms

Menopause symptoms typically reduce on a WFPB diet when there is moderate intake of soy protein. In fact, a recent study has shown that hot flushes can be reduced by up to 84%. *(Barnard, ND; Kahleova, H; Holtz, D et al. The Women's Study for the Alleviation of Vasomotor Symptoms, Menopause Journal, October 2021)*

In my coaching practice, menopause symptoms can be resolved by focusing on eliminating the 'trouble-maker' foods that fuel the Epstein-Barr Virus, such as eggs and dairy products, which are not present in the WFPB diet.

Mental Health

Mental health conditions such as depression, anxiety and unstable moods are strongly connected to the health of our gut, because up to 90% of our serotonin (happy hormone) is produced there.

Brain fog, short term memory loss, concentration problems, vertigo, migraines and headaches also fall under the umbrella of mental health. The Epstein-Barr Virus has a significant role to play here, and I go into greater detail about this in my first book. This virus relies on some of our most common, everyday foods on the SAD diet as its fuel source, leading to symptoms that create these problems. These foods also inflame the vagus nerve, which can lead to vertigo, headaches and migraines. It's important that these foods are removed from the diet to resolve mental health issues, and this is naturally achieved by following a WFPB diet.

Most of my clients have some form of mental health issues when they first come to see me. When we work on fixing the gut and reducing inflammation of the vagus nerve, mental health starts to improve very quickly.

Pain

An awful lot of people live with chronic and unresolved pain. Sometimes pain is caused by muscular or skeletal injury, but for most people, pain is reversible with the removal of inflammatory foods such as dairy products from the diet. Most of my clients have some form of physical pain in the body, and much of the time, it will start to resolve when they start following a plant-based diet.

As an example, my 77-year-old mother suffered from osteo-arthritis for many years and also had a problematic knee. She was initially reluctant to give up dairy-based milk in her daily coffee and baked treats, but eventually she did, and no longer has any arthritic or knee pain whatsoever. As soon as she eats something containing dairy, she gets the 'pins and needles' sensation in her hands and her arthritis flares up.

Sleep

As previously mentioned, the WFPB diet promotes healthy gut bacteria, which then have the important role of helping to produce serotonin. From serotonin, the body produces melatonin, which helps us sleep. Nutrient-dense, whole foods also help the liver perform at its optimum. Many sleep problems have their roots in poor liver function, so when the liver is able to perform its 2,000 functions correctly, it leads to improved sleep.

Stress

There's no doubt that stress is an unavoidable part of life. The problem is, many people are living in a state of constant stress, more commonly known as 'fight or flight', and it's creating some serious health problems. I go into greater detail about addressing the root cause of stress in *From Living Hell to Living Well*, but in the context of this book, food has a major impact on how we experience and respond to stress.

In a nutshell, a dysfunctional gut, inflammation in the body and general poor health exacerbates stress hormones in the body. A WFPB diet promotes great gut health, is anti-inflammatory and creates overall superior health, and is therefore ideal as a means of keeping stress levels in check.

Thyroid

The Adventist Health Study-2 found 50% less prevalence of thyroid problems on a plant-based diet compared with omnivorous diets. *(Tonstad S; Nathan E; Oda K; Fraser GE. Prevalence of hyperthyroidism according to type of vegetarian diet. Public Health Nutrition, 2015)*

However, there are a couple of areas to be mindful of when it comes to a WFPB diet and optimal thyroid health. The first is a risk of iodine deficiency, although only a small amount each day is required in the diet. Iodine can be found in sea vegetables such as arame, dulse, wakame and nori.

Zinc and selenium are also important. You can obtain adequate selenium from one brazil nut per day, while trace amounts can be found in mushrooms and wholegrains.

Weight Loss

A WFPB involves plenty of fibre, which helps to fill you up without additional calories. It also takes the focus away from processed and packaged foods which are usually high in trans-fats. Often, weight loss is something that just happens naturally on a WFPB diet, without having to give it much thought. As long as the bulk of your diet consists of whole, nutrient-dense and fresh foods, excess body fat will naturally fall away. Not only is it great for weight loss, but also for maintaining a stable weight over time.

Blue Zones

I'd like to tell you about a phenomenon that I find absolutely fascinating. There are a series of five regions around the world called the Blue Zones, where the populations have a life expectancy much higher than the global average. These populations have a higher than usual numbers of nonagenarians and centenarians – people who live over the age of 90 and 100 respectively. The five blue zones are in Okinawa, Japan; Sardinia, Italy; Nicoya, Costa Rica; Ikaria, Greece; and Loma Linda, California.

The concept was a result of demographic work by Giovanni Mario Pes, Michael Poulain and Dan Buettner, and the name originated when they drew circles in blue pen around each region on a map.

The purpose of the study was to investigate the reasons why these populations were living longer and healthier lives than other populations around the world. The following commonalities were discovered:

- They follow mostly a plant-based diet, with a focus on local and seasonal produce.
- Intake of fish and meat is low (meat is mainly eaten on special occasions or celebrations and rarely surpasses once per week).
- They eat fewer calories overall.
- There is no smoking and very low intake of alcohol.
- People have healthy social networks with friends and family.
- The people have a strong sense of purpose.
- They get moderate, regular exercise (based around working on the land, gardening, walking cooking, and other daily chores – not a gym in sight!)
- They get plenty of sleep and it's not unusual to take daytime naps.
- They are typically part of religious communities.

An interesting thing about the Blue Zones is that, contrary to the global norm, men do not have a shorter life expectancy than women. The populations in these areas also have around half the rates of chronic disease compared with other western populations, and much fewer cases of dementia. Many of these populations also live in somewhat remote areas and have limited access to health care.

I raise the subject of Blue Zones not just for the plant-based diet component, but because it's a great example of what I mentioned earlier about freedom.

These people are not controlled by food addiction, they are not pummelling their bodies inside a gymnasium, nor are they surviving on too little sleep. They're certainly not counting their calories or downing several glasses of alcohol in the evening.

They are following some fundamental, basic principles for wellbeing, and they are reaping the rewards of long and healthy lives.

Reaching Your Potential

Something I've become aware of and have given a lot of thought to lately is the realisation that living a great (not mediocre) life, achieving our goals and dreams and reaching our full potential has its foundations in excellent health. And for excellent health, we must eat in a way that not only prevents disease but allows our genes to be expressed in the best possible way.

I believe that deep down, everyone wants to live a life of meaning, understand their purpose and strive for the things that make them happy. What makes someone happy will vary from person to person, and I'm not talking about material things. Sure, a flash house and car and regular vacations are lovely to have and there's nothing wrong with wanting those things, but I'm talking about the *intangible* things that lead to a deep sense of contentment.

Things like connections with other people, the satisfaction that comes from contributing to the world around you, the joy in setting yourself a target and reaching it, and the knowledge that you are making the most of your one and precious life.

What I've come to realise is that those deep desires become very difficult to achieve when you don't have great health on your side, because you simply don't have the energy, motivation, willpower and capacity to give them the attention they need to eventuate.

One of my favourite books is *The Magic of Thinking Big*, written by David J Schwartz in 1959. In his book, he talks about living in a world that tries to pull you down Second-Class Street, where narrow thinking and striving to be average is the norm. More people are content to stay on Second-Class Street where it's safe and 'comfortable', than strive to be on First-Class Avenue, which requires one to extend themselves and reach their full potential.

I liken this story to how people approach their health. Most people plod through life without paying much attention to their health, and as a result, they feel average most of the time. They are on Second-Class Street, feeling low on energy, joy and motivation, because their mediocre state of health doesn't allow for anything else. These are generally the people eating the SAD and allowing themselves to be blown whichever way the wind takes them. They end up sick and unsatisfied, feeling like there must be something more but they don't know how to change their lot in life.

The people who reside on First-Class Avenue, on the other hand, are few and far between. These are the ones who take a proactive approach to their health and nip problems in the bud as soon as they arise. They look after their physical, mental and emotional health through good food, exercise, sleep and managing stress. Consequently, they have the stamina and mental capacity to take the required steps to be ambitious and reach their goals.

Please don't misunderstand me. There's nothing wrong with living a quiet and simple life. If that's what brings you contentment and peace, that's wonderful! But if you're someone who knows you're capable of more, yet unsure of how to get to where you want to be, it might be time to take a closer look at your state of health.

I use myself as an example in this instance. I can look back a few years ago, before I took my diet and lifestyle in hand and can see that I was plodding. I had a good job with the local council which I liked (but didn't love), became a full-time mum, and had a simple and relatively stress-free lifestyle.

I definitely wasn't unhappy by any means, but I knew on a deeper level that I had more in me. I had no idea what that 'more' was, but it was there, and in fact it had always been there, since about the age of 18. That's when I knew I had a strong interest in anything associated with personal growth and development and realised I was in charge of my destiny.

When I got sick, my confidence plummeted, and I felt very lost. Those couple of years were all about survival and just getting through each day. But when my health started to turn a corner and I came out the other side, I realised that my new-found plant-based diet was starting to transform my life. Not only was my body healing, it was starting to thrive.

I noticed my mind was clear, energy levels were soaring, and I felt like I was skipping, not dragging my feet through the days. In the evenings, I wasn't collapsing on the couch to binge-watch Netflix with a bar of chocolate. I was too busy getting curious and starting to ask some bigger questions of myself.

What did I really want to do? What was I capable of? What were my bucket list items? Would I be satisfied if I never achieved them?

Suddenly I had the strong desire, and more importantly, the *ability* to start tapping into that 'something more' I knew was inside.

Today, I witness the same thing with my clients. When they first come to see me, they're usually in pretty bad shape. They are barely able to cope with the basics of life, let alone find the desire or motivation to tap into their 'more'. Once they start following the plant-based diet and their health improves, the light switches on and their whole energy shifts. It's magnificent to see and reconfirms to me over and over again that the plant-based lifestyle can be utterly life-changing.

Another interesting thing happens when you begin to experience great health. You start noticing on a deeper level what's happening with the people around you, particularly those who are coming into their 40s, 50s and beyond. You'll start to see a significant number of people who are tired, drawn, stressed, overweight and generally unhappy – in other words, suffering the effects of mediocre or poor health. You find yourself in conversations about their aches and pains, unwanted fat rolls and all the horrible things about getting older. You empathise with their struggles but know it doesn't have to be that way.

You begin to realise that while everyone else is starting to fall apart, you are just starting to live. And with that cracking piece of knowledge under your belt, something spectacular happens.

Life takes off and you start stepping into the person you were born to be.

Digging up the Dirt

Are you on First-Class Avenue or Second-Class Street with your health? What particular health issues are you struggling with and how are they holding you back from reaching your potential? What does this mean for your future?

_____

_____

_____

_____

_____

_____

_____

_____

_____

_____

_____

_____

_____

_____

CHAPTER SIX
Setting the Scene

If you've come this far, hopefully you are starting to appreciate what all the fuss is about with the WFPB diet – and why I've dedicated months of my life to writing about it!

Even though a lot can be communicated through the written or spoken word, sometimes I wish I could take someone who is struggling with their health and perhaps feeling hesitant about the plant-based diet and put them inside the body of someone who does eat this way. That sounds strange, I know, but hear me out.

I want people to understand what it's like to go from a very sick person – I'm talking about wanting to curl-up-and-die-type-sick – to a person who experiences incredible health every single day. I want them to understand how the wellspring of vitality and contentment that resides inside a healthy body can completely and utterly transform a person's life. I want them to grasp the concept of what it's like to be able to navigate the rollercoaster of life by supporting their body and mind in the best possible way.

I am that person who wanted to curl up and die with poor health, by the way. However, I came out the other side and realised there was a whole world waiting for me. Not only was it waiting, but it was also *available* to me, because I had the health to pursue it. It had nothing to do with good timing or good fortune, and everything to do with inviting plant foods into my life.

My point is, I could write a hundred books on the subject, but for you to experience what I did, you must try it for yourself. That's the only way to truly understand how your life can be transformed as a result.

My wish for you is that you adopt this way of life and never look back. But for that to happen, there's a few things to be aware of that can derail your progress. The last thing I want is for you to try, fail, then throw your hands up in exasperation and say, *"nah, that didn't work."*

It's also important to be aware of what will help you succeed, and these are the things to direct your attention towards and leverage as much as possible.

This chapter is all about helping you become someone who embraces positive change and sticks with it, because in reality, many people can't, or won't do this over the long term, even when their current situation is untenable.

But you're not that person, right? You're ready to take action!

Setting the Scene

Overcoming Obstacles

A lot of people hear the words 'vegan' or 'plant-based' or 'no meat' and immediately side-line the idea as too difficult, undesirable or 'fluffy and new-agey' – without even giving it a chance. I get it; it's a lot to wrap one's head around.

Changing ingrained behaviours and habits we've carried for decades can be challenging and uncomfortable to say the least. Moving towards the unknown takes a certain level of commitment, motivation and willpower that can be tricky to muster.

Each person's motivating factors for change are unique and individual to them, but a common theme we see in our coaching practice is people who are so sick that they *absolutely must* make a change. Their health has spiralled so far downwards that not taking action could spell debilitation or death at worst, or a joyless existence at best.

> *"Change is painful, but nothing is as painful as staying stuck somewhere you don't belong."*
>
> (Mandy Hale)

Discarding old patterns and habits is fundamental to reaching the goal of optimal health, but there are a couple of hurdles that can derail the process. These are related to conflicting goals and our ego.

Conflicting Goals

This is where a person wants two things that conflict with each other. For example, they want to lose weight, but they also want to eat junk food. Or they know they should go to bed earlier to improve their sleep, but they also want to stay up late watching movies on Netflix.

Something I talk about a lot with my clients is the crucial process of identifying their 'why' or 'driving force' before they embark on a new goal. Without being crystal clear on their reasons for wanting to change, they are likely to stumble when the going gets tough.

Your 'why' can't be vague. It must punch at the very heart of your deepest desires, where not following through will create a great deal of pain.

> *"People will do more to avoid pain,*
> *than they will to gain pleasure."*
>
> (Tony Robbins)

In other words, avoiding painful situations will always trump seeking out pleasurable situations.

Your 'why' must evoke a strong feeling of pain if you don't take action. For example, the pain of not losing weight must outweigh the pleasure of eating junk food. The pain of waking up feeling exhausted must outweigh the pleasure of staying up late.

Along this vein, I like to ask my clients to imagine themselves in 12 months' time if they don't follow through. What is your life like? Can you live with the consequences of not taking action? Are you prepared to continue with the status quo? The key is to drill down deeply into your pain points and identify the reason why failure simply isn't an option.

Bingo! That is your 'why'.

And when you find it, the dilemma of conflicting goals evaporates. The pain of not losing weight is so immense, that the pleasure of eating junk food isn't even on the radar.

When you think about your 'why' for transitioning to a plant-based diet, something like 'because it sounds good' is not enough. This will not keep you on track when something happens to derail your progress. *"Because my family members drop dead in their 50s from heart disease and I don't want that to happen to me"* is much more powerful. The pain of a premature death outweighs the pleasure of not taking action and remaining comfortable with your existing, unhealthy eating patterns.

Self-Image and Ego

As humans, we get tied up in knots thinking about how other people perceive us, and our behaviour can be influenced by this. From a biological standpoint, this is about raising esteem or status to increase the odds of survival.

Our ego wants us to succeed, and we use our imagination to picture what life could be like if we do. But our ego can also create our downfall when expectations become too high and there is a risk of failure. For us to preserve esteem and status, we would rather sabotage ourselves and hold on to the illusion that 'things could be great if only I'd tried' – rather than try our best and fail. The tragic consequence of this is we never end up realising our potential.

This can be a reason why you see some people constantly yo-yoing with their health, particularly when it comes to weight loss. They will be gung-ho with a new healthy eating plan, are fully committed and start seeing great results, then they sabotage themselves because they are scared of what will happen if they try, but still fail. This is usually a subconscious pattern they aren't even aware of. This then becomes a vicious cycle which is repeated time and time again, and the only result is they end up stuck and frustrated, and often say things like, *"Nothing ever works for me."*

The key learning here is to resist setting expectations that are too high or unrealistic. When you allow yourself some room to fall out of line occasionally, the chances of overall success are actually much higher. This is why I encourage my clients to follow my coaching plan at about 80-90%. Setting expectations at 100% creates far too much pressure and will inevitably end in failure and frustration.

It's important to focus on progress rather than perfection. Mistakes or mis-steps should be viewed as opportunities to learn, rather than failures.

Any goal relating to health should also be set to a realistic time frame. Our 1-1 coaching programmes have a 6-12 week duration, but the ultimate goal is to teach people how to adopt sensible, sustainable changes over the long term.

I always encourage my clients to give themselves some leeway when it comes to transitioning to a plant-based diet. Craving some meat? Have it. Want an ice cream? Have it. Just pick and choose your moments wisely. I don't believe in deprivation and making things difficult, and neither should you!

Setting the Scene

Preparing for Success

Now we are aware of a few of the things that can result in failure, let's investigate the things that will determine whether you will be successful in your health-related goals.

The first is if your 'why' is powerful enough, which we've already discussed.

Another is whether you feel you have the ability, knowledge and skills necessary to succeed.

Transitioning to a plant-based diet is a fairly significant life change and can be tricky and confusing if you don't know where to start. Personally, I did it on my own, simply because I was chronically ill and I had a super-strong 'why' – the pain of not getting better outweighed the pleasure of lying on the couch and eating unhealthy food! I also didn't have anyone to teach me the ropes, aside from a few different people sharing their experiences and recipes through books, podcasts and YouTube.

I really could have used someone like myself to give me meal plans, grocery lists and recipes to follow! This is the exact reason I decided to study plant-based nutrition and share my knowledge and first-hand experience with people. I knew there would be a demand for this type of coaching, and I wasn't wrong.

When you have someone walking alongside you, guiding you in the right direction and keeping you accountable, your chances of success are so much greater.

A third factor for success is identifying a goal you know you can achieve that will lead you towards a community that is important to you or that you care about. We are social beings who thrive on a sense of belonging and being part of something 'bigger than ourselves' can be a great motivator.

Everyone's reasons for going plant-based will be different, but a big part of the plant-based movement is about connecting with a tribe of other like-minded people. There are vegans whose first priority might be animal welfare or environmental impacts, and they love being part of the 'bigger picture' to initiate change, even though their personal contribution might seem like a drop in the ocean.

The main thing to consider is whether your goal and the community you would like to be part of aligns with your personal values and whether you feel it's a good fit for you.

Lastly, we can't forget the importance of finding your support crew. These are the people who are going to support and encourage you, pick you up when you fall over, keep you accountable and give you a kick up the backside when necessary.

Your cheerleaders won't necessarily be the people you expect. You may find that your close friends and family aren't really that fussed on supporting you with your goals, and this can be for lots of different reasons. Maybe they're not on your wavelength with this particular goal, or they have different priorities or things going on in their own lives they are focused on.

If your best friend is going to give you a hard time for 'not getting enough protein' and doesn't support your choice to stop eating meat, he or she is not your support crew. If the colleague you get along well with is going to laugh at you when you choose not to have a scone with jam and cream at morning tea, they are not your support crew, either.

Setting the Scene

Don't take it personally if someone you expected to encourage you, doesn't. Instead, seek out the people who will be happy to walk beside you on the journey and give you the support you need.

Even if you can't find someone in your immediate circle who fits the bill, don't be afraid to seek out like-minded people online. There is a whole world wide web full of people looking to connect with others every single day. Start googling or searching on Facebook to find the groups you want to be part of, then join them and participate! I personally do this because I don't have a large circle of people around me in my everyday life who follow a plant-based diet – yet!

Don't feel like you have to rely on your immediate friends and family to encourage you with making positive changes in your life. These days, it is so easy to connect with people over the other side of the globe who will be more than happy to support you. Those who are interested in your goals and are genuinely happy to see you achieve them are the ones you want in your corner.

Side-Stepping Trends

Something I like to distance myself and my clients from are fads and trends. They have no place in our coaching practice, nor do I waste my time delving into them to find what the hype is all about. I know for sure that fads and trends simply don't work. As soon as I hear the words, *"The new trend taking the world by storm"*, I switch off.

There are so many 'trendy' diet plans out there, and sadly, they are everything to do with generating profit, and nothing to do with your health. The sooner you can accept this, the better off you'll be.

Firstly, there's the Standard American Diet (SAD) which we've already touched on. This isn't so much a trend, but a way of life for most people. This is a diet high in animal fat, protein and saturated fat, low in fresh fruits and vegetables, fibre and complex carbohydrates, and is highly processed.

In a nutshell, the SAD has created a global health and environmental catastrophe.

Then there are other so-called 'healthy' diet plans, such as *Weight Watchers*, *Jenny Craig*, *Paleo*, *Atkins*, *Ketogenic* and *Mediterranean*. Each one differs in terms of what to include, avoid and limit. They range from omnivore-based (plant and animal origin), to semi-vegetarian/flexitarian (plant-based with some animal products), to pesco-vegetarian (plant-based with fish, dairy and eggs) to vegetarian/lacto-ovo (plants, dairy, eggs) to vegan (excludes all animal products).

Many of us have probably attempted one or more of these in the past – I certainly have! – and perhaps you still follow one of them. Don't get me wrong – some of these diets have some really great parts to them, such as watching portion sizes (Weight Watchers) or avoiding sugars and alcohol (Paleo/Atkins).

But there are also some not-so-good parts with all of these diets which must be highlighted – not as a criticism, but to bring awareness to the dangers and long-term consequences of following them. Let's take a look at a few examples.

Weight Watchers

Weight Watchers places an emphasis on 'everything in moderation' and endorses plenty of fresh fruits and vegetables. Nothing is off limits, but calories and portion sizes are carefully controlled. Each type of food is allocated 'points' and you must stick to your allocated number of points per day. Sounds okay, right?

Well, let's assume you are allowed 30 points per day, and a large chunk of chocolate cake equates to 15 of those points. You eat the cake, and this means you only have 15 points left to 'spend' on food for the rest of the day. This might mean that you skip lunch or dinner, or maybe you find something that is worth 15 points, such as two pieces of toast with lashings of butter and jam, and a jumbo sugary cappuccino. Of course, a couple of pieces of fruit and some vegetables would be a better option, but not everyone is going to take this path when there might be yummier foods to spend their points on.

Does a piece of chocolate cake, two pieces of buttery toast and a sweet, milky drink sound like a balanced diet? Sure, you may lose some weight by sticking to the points system, but you certainly won't be giving your body the nutrition it desperately needs.

Weight loss does not automatically equate to great long-term health.

Ketogenic Diet

Let's look at the Keto diet. This one is very popular at the moment. I could tell you about all the ex-Keto clients we see who are in bad shape mentally and physically but needless to say, that's a book in itself!

The problem with the Keto diet is that it focuses on high amounts of protein (particularly animal protein, which automatically equates to high fat). It also limits carbohydrates, which is disastrous for the adrenal system because it then has to compensate for the lack of fuel (glucose) by releasing stress hormones such as adrenaline and cortisol to keep the body safe and able to perform not only its everyday functions, but to keep up with your busy schedule.

High levels of saturated fat in the diet thickens the blood, which means the heart must work harder to pump thick, sludgy blood around the body. Not only this, but the liver also has to work extra hard to break down the excess fats in the body, slowing it down and making it sluggish, stagnant and sick. Then there's the issue of excess meat stripping away essential stomach acids and creating all sorts of mess in the gut.

Low-carb diets might work in the short term when it comes to weight loss, but so does drug and alcohol addiction. It doesn't mean it's healthy! There is also no compelling evidence to suggest that high protein, low-carb diets have long-term health benefits.

Paleo

The Paleolithic diet subscribes to the notion that our ancestors ate plenty of meat and very few grains and legumes, so this way of eating must be healthy. In actual fact, meat was very sparse because the only way it could be obtained was through hunting. Our ancestors were actually largely herbivorous (plant-based), and for the majority of human evolution, cholesterol was almost non-detectable in the diet, which indicates that meat was not nearly as prevalent as we think.

In recent years, the Paleo diet has been strongly linked with the sport of CrossFit. A study was undertaken among 43 young, healthy cross-fitters who were put on a Paleo diet. After 10 weeks, their LDL cholesterol ('bad' cholesterol) increased, while their HDL cholesterol ('good' cholesterol) decreased. *(Physicians Committee for Responsible Medicine: Paleo Diet Leads to Worsening Cholesterol, International Journal of Exercise Science, 2014)*

Vegetarian

A vegetarian diet includes fruits, vegetables, whole grains, legumes, dairy and eggs, while avoiding meat and fish. At the crux of it, this type of diet isn't really much different from a meat-eater's because it's still high in dairy, refined flour and oils - none of which are good for long-term health.

Vegan

Remember in Chapter One I mentioned it's possible to be a junk food vegan? This can be the case not only with rubbish foods like *Coca Cola* and *Oreos*, but also if you replace meat and other animal products with things like highly processed fake meats, too much oil, or refined plant fragments processed into snack foods. A healthy vegan diet is one that focuses on mainly plant-based foods.

There are many other diets out there that claim to be cure-alls and many of them have some good redeeming features. But it always pays to remember that these diets are all about generating profit for the manufacturers and marketers. Their claims from a health perspective are often wishy-washy and not evidence-based, and fancy marketing tactics can over-ride common sense.

Full o' Beans!

The thing I love about the WFPB diet is that it's not a trend. It's a sensible, sustainable approach to eating fresh, whole, nutrient-dense foods provided by nature that give the body the absolute best chance for optimal health and wellbeing.

If you need even more convincing, I highly recommend watching some well-known documentaries[4] that will reinforce much of what is in this book, with some additional 'holy cow' moments in there, too! *Forks over Knives*, *The Gamechangers*, and *What the Health* are great ones to start with, and there's plenty more out there when you're done with those!

---

[4]*Please see the 'Further Viewing' section at the back of the book for more information.*

Setting the Scene

Digging up the Dirt

What is your 'why' for changing the way you eat? Remember your 'why' has to create pain if you don't follow through.
In setting yourself up for success, which obstacles do you need to overcome?

_____

_____

_____

_____

_____

_____

_____

_____

_____

_____

_____

_____

CHAPTER SEVEN
Practice is Power

We've now reached the super fun part of the book, where we get into the exciting details of how to put this wonderful new way of life into practice. There's a lot to learn, but rest assured it will all be broken down into easy-to-swallow bite-size pieces – pun intended!

Only you can decide how committed you will be to the WFPB lifestyle. Some people transition more slowly than others, but if you're in not-so-great shape physically and mentally or your goal is to reverse pre-existing health conditions, it's often best to transition fully and quickly – with a bit of wriggle room, of course.

Following this lifestyle is easier than you might think.

But, that doesn't mean you won't face some curveballs and challenges along the way. Changing the way you eat comes from changing your behaviour and figuring out how you will maintain focus and motivation. And as we've already learnt, if you want to attain your goal of optimal health, you will also need to discard some old habits, dependencies, addictions and mindsets.

This chapter is all about providing you with the basics of what you need to know to begin following a WFPB lifestyle. I could talk until the plant-based cows come home about this (it's my favourite subject after all!) but at the end of the day, we learn best by taking action and doing. This information is intended to get you started, so you then have the confidence to go and try it for yourself.

Firstly, let's pause for a moment and go back to your 'why'. Remember, you must be very clear on your driving force for why you want to change your diet in the first place. Once you've identified it, you are far more likely to follow through over the long term, as opposed to starting with a hiss and a roar because it's the next new thing, only to find yourself going off the rails when you hit a speed bump.

Here are some of the key areas that will set you up for success:

Meal Planning

In the beginning, you will need to come up with something resembling a plan, because as we know, those who fail to plan, plan to fail! Planning your meals will prevent you from reaching for the nearest cookie or meat-lovers pizza when you've had a busy day or just can't be bothered to cook.

These are a few tips to set you up for success when planning your meals:

Practice is Power

- Prepare a menu for the week – this will ensure you are organised and will save you time and money.
- Choose easy and familiar recipes to start with – e.g. salads or rice and beans. For your favourite recipes that contain meat such as lasagne, tacos or chilli, replace with a plant-based option – i.e. faux chicken, faux mince or tofu.
- Explore plant-based recipes that interest you in cookbooks or online and have fun experimenting with new flavours.
- Try restaurants with plant-based options on the menu. These days, most cafes and restaurants offer these options. Get a feel for the types of foods you can order when you go out for a meal.
- If you are techy minded, start searching online for helpful websites or apps to help you, such as recipe organisation (PaprikaApp); menu planning (happyherbivore.com); or the Forks Over Knives menu planner app.
- Create a master grocery list of all the new types of foods you come across in recipes.
- Think about batch cooking, where you prepare the week's meals in advance, for example on a Sunday.
- Think about who can help you prepare meals, such as your spouse or children.
- Enlist the support of a plant-based specialist (me!) who will set you up with meal plans, grocery lists and recipes to remove all the guess work and make it super easy!

Shopping Secrets

When you go to the supermarket, pay attention to where all the fresh food is. You will see it situated mainly around the perimeter of the store. Then, go down the aisles and look at what's there. Cardboard boxes, plastic bottles and a swathe of other packaging will greet you with bright and shiny labels, enticing you to buy. It all looks lovely and inviting, but it's mostly processed junk full of artificial flavourings, colourings, additives and preservatives that will weaken your immune system and make you sick. This is where the saying, *"Stick to the perimeter and avoid the aisles"* comes from.

Here are some key items to look for and things to keep in mind at the supermarket:

- Most of your food should come from the fresh fruit and vegetable section. If you want ease and convenience, you can also buy pre-chopped vegetables, but these are often more expensive and in environmentally unfriendly packaging.
- Frozen fruits and vegetables are also an excellent option as they are convenient and full of vitamins, nutrients and antioxidants.
- Steer clear of anything in the frozen section that is not fruit or vegetables.[5]
- Beware of the section labelled 'Natural Foods' or similar. This is a marketing trick and while there are certainly some great, healthy foods in this area, there's also a lot of processed and packaged foods, too. Be sure to read the labels.
- Choose whole grains such as 100% wholegrain pasta, rice and oats, or gluten-free varieties such as millet, buckwheat, or quinoa.
- Choose low or no sodium varieties of canned beans and vegetables.
- Be careful with boxed cereals as these are often extremely high in sugar. Look for wholegrain/low sugar or gluten-free

---

[5] When you are transitioning to a WFPB lifestyle, it is fine to use faux meats as meat replacements. These are not recommended to be used regularly or long-term, however, because they can be highly processed.

varieties. Oats are your best choice for a healthy breakfast cereal.
- Read labels on packaged sauces because many are full of sugar, salt and fat.
- Shop in the bulk food section but aim for natural, raw and unsalted.
- Watch out for snack foods which are usually loaded with fat, salt and sugar.
- Herbs and spices are wonderful staples on a plant-based diet and great varieties can be found in health shops or ethnic markets.

As I mentioned in my first book, one of the best things I did to educate myself on healthy foods was to take some time to wander through the aisles of the supermarket. I studied nutritional labels and became familiar with what the numbers and letters on the labels mean. I highly recommend you do the same so you can approach food shopping with knowledge and confidence.

Bang For Your Buck

There is the belief that following a plant-based diet is expensive, but actually fresh, unprocessed food is far more affordable than processed and packaged food. The key is to be as organised as possible and pay attention to which shops in your local area will provide the best value for money.

Here are some ways to stretch your dollar further:

- Buy locally produced and seasonal food (also ensure it is pesticide and GMO free).

- If you do choose packaged foods, look for less than five ingredients on the label (you are paying for all those nasty additives!)
- Do meal prep on the weekends, such as cooking a batch of rice, cooking legumes or chopping vegetables to use up food that might otherwise go to waste.
- Cook enough to freeze portions for future use so you always have something on hand when you can't or don't want to cook – so you don't resort to ordering takeaways!
- Prepare extra quantities at dinner time to have for lunch the next day.
- Purchase vegetables whole rather than pre-chopped.
- Vegetables (especially leafy greens) should be a priority if you're on a budget because they offer the greatest health benefits.
- Buy in bulk.
- Farmers markets are a great place to find organic and inexpensive fresh produce.
- Consider joining a local co-op for cheaper produce.
- Avoid bottled juices, flavoured water and tea as they are often loaded with sugar and empty calories.
- Aim not to waste food by planning meals in advance.
- If you can, find friends and/or neighbours who you can trade home-grown fruits and vegetables with.
- Meals such as soups and casseroles are very filling, go a long way and are inexpensive to make.
- Sometimes you can buy fruit that is about to go off (such as bananas) very cheaply. Freeze for smoothies and ice creams. Do the same for fresh fruit at home that is about to go bad.

Practice is Power

Batch Cooking

This is a great option if you don't enjoy the cooking process or are often running short on time. You can prepare all of the week's meals on one day or cook up large batches of staples such as potatoes, legumes or rice all at once. Another option is to double or triple recipes, so you only have to cook once every few days.

Here are some batch cooking suggestions:

- Cook a large batch of grains such as rice, millet and quinoa to make casseroles, veggie burgers, soups or to top with beans and veggies. Experiment with different types a few times a week and freeze leftovers for later use.
- Cook a large batch of beans such as chickpeas, lentils, pinto or black beans. Speed up the process by using an instant pot or pressure cooker, and freeze leftovers for later use.
- Make a large pot of soup. Soup is a one-pot meal and is very easy to prepare. Experiment with a different type of soup each week.
- Chilli is very versatile and can be eaten in many different ways, such as by itself, on top of potatoes, over homemade tortilla chips, over grains, or in a Buddha bowl (see my recipe in Chapter Ten).
- Double or triple the recipe for burger patties and freeze for later use. It's best to freeze the patties after they've been cooked so they don't fall apart in the freezer.
- Bake potatoes in bulk then use them in different meals during the week, such as with steamed veggies or chilli.

Here is an example of how you can take one 'staple' (brown rice), cook it in a large batch then use it over a week:

Monday: Serve rice with chilli beans and a side salad for a quick, easy and nutritious meal.

Tuesday: Use rice as a base in a tortilla and top with cooked legumes, veggies and vegan aioli.

Wednesday: Stir fry rice in a pan with soy sauce and veggies, topped with sesame seeds.

Thursday: Try using rice instead of pasta with an Alfredo or Marinara sauce.

Friday: Have a breakfast of warm rice, oat milk, cinnamon and fresh fruit.

Useful Tools and Utensils

It's likely that you already have most of what you need to cook great plant-based meals. If you plan to adopt this lifestyle long-term, here are a few excellent tools to invest in. Keep in mind that your needs will depend on what type of cook you are. If you are someone who loves to spend time in the kitchen and come up with all sorts of flavourful concoctions, your appliance/utensil needs will be much greater than someone who prefers making quick, no-fuss meals.

- A high-powered blender such as a *Vitamix*. These are pricey but absolutely worth the investment because they have very powerful blades and a 10-year guarantee. A *Vitamix* is fantastic for making soups, ice cream, smoothies, sauces and dressings. I bought mine almost immediately when I transitioned to a WFPB diet and it's been the best investment I could have

made. Every member of my household uses it at least once per day.[6]
- An immersion (stick) blender can be useful for things like basic smoothies or milkshakes but probably not necessary if you have a more powerful blender.
- A pressure cooker can save time by reducing cooking times by up to 50%, while retaining nutrients.
- Food processor
- Garlic press
- Zester
- Spiraliser
- Juicer.

If you can track down a local store that supplies kitchen tools to restaurants, you may be able to get some great deals on basic kitchen supplies.

Say 'No' to Oil

Cooking oils are often marketed as 'heart healthy', but they're actually anything but. They're basically pure fat that will hijack your liver and clog up your arteries.

If you are currently suffering from ill health, I recommend you learn how to cook without oil. If you feel relatively healthy, this is still a great goal to aim for. It's simple when you know how and once you start, you will wonder why you ever needed to use oil in the first place!

---

[6] Beware of cheaper blenders. Their blades are weaker, and you will likely end up having to replace them (or the whole appliance) if you are wanting to make smoothie bowls/ice creams because they will burn out. I learned this one the hard way by having to continuously replace my blender. In the end, I bit the bullet and invested in a *Vitamix*. If you are lucky, you may be able to find a second-hand *Vitamix*, but this can be tricky because I doubt many people would part with them once they realise how amazing they are!

Invest in non-stick cookware, such as heavy-bottomed stainless-steel pans, enamel coated cast iron, or ceramic titanium. Silicone ovenware and parchment (baking) paper are also safe options for baking, roasting vegetables and preparing desserts.

A simple way to cook without oil is to warm your pan on a medium heat, then add onions to sauté. Onions have their own essential oils to grease the pan, and you can use a splash of cooking wine, vegetable broth or water if the onions start to stick.

Let's Go Out!

Dining out can bring a whole new challenge to following a WFPB diet, and my advice is just to do your best. Just because a restaurant may offer vegan or plant-based options, they won't always be healthy if they use highly processed ingredients or are saturated with oil.

Have you ever been seated at a restaurant table with someone who starts to nit-pick the menu with the waiter? They want their meal to be vegan, with no oil, dressing strictly on the side, no nuts, and absolutely no 'fake-cheese'. Don't get me wrong, there's nothing bad about knowing what you like to eat and being strict about it, and most eating establishments will do their best to accommodate you. But in my experience, picking apart the menu to make sure everything is perfect is a really difficult way to live.

When I first went plant-based, I made a promise to myself that I wouldn't be 'that person' who made my own or someone else's life hard because I was super-strict about my diet. These days, I take a more relaxed approach when I am out for dinner at a restaurant or someone's house. I do my best with the choices available, then go with the flow. So what if I eat a bit of something I wouldn't normally eat? It's not the end of the world.

Of course, this will come down to personal preference about how strict you wish to be, but there's nothing worse than watching a tense exchange between a waiter and customer who expects perfection and then complains if it's not right.

Here are some tips to help you find healthy choices when you go out for a meal:

- Be prepared by checking the menu online in advance so you know what to order.
- Know what to look for when it comes to healthy/not-so-healthy options. Look for the words 'steamed', 'baked' or 'grilled' which generally means the meal is prepared without oil. Avoid the words 'fried', 'rich', 'creamy' or 'crispy' which usually mean high fat and high oil.
- Ask for oil-free meals (this isn't always possible).
- Ask for brown rice instead of white.
- Ask for non-dairy based sauces and no cheese.
- Ask for dressings on the side.
- Don't be afraid to ask for substitute dishes (for example, steamed rice instead of creamy potatoes).
- Ask for wholegrain bread instead of white, or even better, gluten free.

Above all, don't try to be perfect. Enjoy your meal, even if it's not what you had originally planned or wanted. The important thing is progress, not perfection.

Getting the Family on Board

It's not always easy to get other members of the family on board when it comes to serving plant-based meals, especially if they're not used to it or have eaten a lot of meat or dairy products in the past. The key is to be patient, and not expect miracles overnight.

When I transitioned to a plant-based diet, my husband Steve was very understanding because I was very sick, and he wanted to support me in getting better. Steve had always been a devoted meat eater and would eat it every day, and sometimes multiple times per day. I knew that telling him I didn't want to cook it anymore was a big call, and I'm really fortunate he was encouraging. I realise that not all spouses react in this way, because my clients tell me so.

However, more often than not, when other family members are introduced to plant-based meals, they are pleasantly surprised at how tasty and filling they can be. A lot of people have the misconception that being plant-based is all about only eating 'rabbit food' like lettuce and salads, but this is far from accurate. It's very common for the spouse to be sceptical at first, but they soon change their mind when they realise they can have a delicious and satisfying meal that doesn't contain meat or lashings of cheese or butter. And of course, there's nothing stopping them having a bit of meat on the side.

Kids can present another challenge, particularly if they are picky eaters. It can be frustrating to get them to try new foods, but the more they see a certain food or experience a certain taste, the more they will accept that it's just part of life and their tastebuds will start to adjust. This can take time, so hang in there and don't be concerned if it seems like an uphill battle you'll never win. Gradually, you will notice them start to eat these new foods without question

Practice is Power

and they'll soon be gobbling down a bowl of Chickpea Curry in five minutes flat – check out my recipe in Chapter Ten!

As I mentioned, my kids are roughly 80% plant-based. I find this works well because it allows room for them to enjoy time with their grandparents or friends and have some of the foods they love, such as a chocolate ice cream or cheesy corn chips. Frankly, I don't have the desire to worry about what they are eating 24/7 and I don't want them to feel deprived to the point that they develop an unhealthy relationship with 'forbidden' foods later in life.

There are no hard and fast rules around what you should do when it comes to feeding your family, so take some time to see how things evolve and what works best. Expect there to be some trial and error and screwed up faces, and trust that it does get easier.

Kids tend to appreciate their food more when they are involved in the cooking process. Here are some simple ways to include them and help them develop their skills:

- Tearing up lettuce or spinach leaves for salads.
- Using measuring cups and spoons.
- Washing fruit and vegetables.
- Crumbling food, such as tofu.
- Snapping beans/broccoli/cauliflower florets.
- Scooping or mashing.
- Spreading with the back of a spoon.
- Sprinkling herbs and spices.
- Arranging toppings, such as on pizza/porridge.

Rejigging Your Food Environment

Your food environment is influenced by a number of different factors that decide what, where, why, how and when you eat. This is important to understand so you can be aware and proactive about making good decisions when you transition to a plant-based diet.

Here are some helpful ways to set you up for success:

- Bring a healthy lunch and snacks to work so you're not tempted by takeaways or vending machines.
- Don't be shy about asking for healthier options at the staff café.
- Join forces with a friend or colleague and make a deal to bring healthy food to work, and keep each other accountable.
- Request a special meal if you're going to a work event (vegan/ gluten-free etc).
- Come prepared to social gatherings by bringing a plant-based dish to share.
- Be honest with your host about what you can eat and offer to contribute.
- Find local cafes or restaurants that serve a variety of food options so you can suggest somewhere to go with friends or family.

From my own experience, I have realised that the ease (or not) of transitioning to plant-based diet is based 80% around mindset. When I was very sick and desperate to get better, I was 100% committed because I wanted so badly to be well again.

There are no rules around how you should or shouldn't undertake the process. Some people want to fully embrace the lifestyle overnight. Others take longer because they want to figure out whether it will work for them. Trust yourself and do what feels right for you. And whether you tell yourself it will be easy or difficult, you will be right!

Socialising

You are potentially going to come up against a few social challenges on your plant-based journey, but they don't have to be a big deal. I like to refer to social challenges as 'social opportunities' because as I've mentioned, mindset is a big part of this.

For many people, the transition to a plant-based lifestyle can feel more daunting than it actually is because of the social aspect. It can take time and practice to learn how to manage the intentions and opinions of others.

Years ago, when I was researching the plant-based diet, I came across an article written by author and plant-based advocate, Kathy Freston, who wrote about the types of social challenges she encountered when she first went plant-based. I'm so glad I read it, because interestingly, I have encountered many of these situations in some shape or form and her suggestions on how to deal with them with confidence and grace have been very useful. The information below has been adapted from Kathy's article, with a few of my own suggestions thrown in, too!

Responding to Negativity

Let's say a friend wants to remind you of how important protein is and that you will surely succumb to osteoporosis if you don't get enough calcium. Or they bring your attention to a 'scientific' article about how humans were designed to be carnivores and the worst possible thing you could do is to just eat plants – trust me, this stuff does happen!

A plant-based diet or veganism is often dismissed as a 'fad' or 'extreme' because it challenges society's commonly held belief that animal protein is essential in the diet. Followers of this way of life can come up against comments such as, *"Are you still doing that vegan thing?"*, as if surely, it's only a matter of time before you come to your senses!

Make sure you have a couple of simple, well-founded quotes up your sleeve as a response, such as, *"Even the Heart Foundation is recognising that a plant-based diet is healthy and that followers of this lifestyle have overall superior health."*

I also like to refer people to books written by various doctors such as *The China Study* by Dr T Colin Campbell or *How Not to Die* by Dr Michael Greger about how to prevent and reverse disease.

When Meat is Pushed on You

If a friend refuses to take no for an answer when you refuse meat off the barbeque, reply with something like, *"Well, there's a lot of heart disease in my family and there's so much evidence now about the link between heart disease and meat that I'm not willing to take the risk."*

Referring to evidence and facts is a good way to stop a potential argument in its tracks, and don't be surprised if all of a sudden, your friend develops a newfound interest in your diet.

In the early days – while you are still coming to grips with your new way of eating – plant-based meat and dairy replacement products can help to ease friction in social settings. For example, at a party you can throw your 'sausages' or 'beef patties' on the barbeque with everyone else. These types of replacement foods can actually help to make plant-based eating more 'normal', because other people can see that you can still eat things that look the same and have a similar taste as regular meat.

Ethical Arguments

People who call themselves 'vegan' can sometimes find themselves in the thick of difficult conversations. For example, you are out with friends and discussing your reasons for being vegan. You explain that you don't like the thoughts of what happens to animals in the process of becoming food and it doesn't feel right to eat them anymore. Your friend then asks, *"So, why are you wearing a leather jacket?"* Don't get defensive or feel guilty, rather just explain that you are doing your best for now and one day you plan to no longer wear any products associated with animals.

Awkward Gifts

You recently did a kind deed for a new friend and they thank you with a gift basket of salami and cheese. One option is to thank them for their kindness while being honest about not eating animal products. This way you are making your preferences clear from the outset and there won't be any confusion later on.

Another option is to graciously accept the gift and pass it on to someone who will appreciate it. The danger here is that your new friend will be none-the-wiser, and you will likely find yourself having to explain your eating preferences further down the track, for example, when they ask you over for dinner.

Feeling Unsupported

If your family or friends take umbrage at your new lifestyle or make it clear they don't agree with it, be strong and remember their comments aren't really about you. Often when we change our habits or preferences for the better, people close to us can feel threatened because their own shortcomings are highlighted. Don't take it personally and remain confident in your choices. This can take practice, especially if you feel hurt that they aren't trying harder to be understanding or supportive. In time, you will come to accept that their opinions don't need to have any bearing on yours.

Feeling Isolated

At some point you may end up feeling 'on the outer' if other people around you don't share your views or values. Significant changes or defining moments in life can emphasise where existing relationships may have run their course or lost their spark.

Transitioning to a plant-based diet is an indicator that you are on the path of self-improvement, and sometimes it can feel like others around you aren't on that path. If you're feeling isolated or misunderstood, you may need to change your social circle, and this isn't necessarily a bad thing. When you find the people who gel with you and your goals, you are encouraged to shine and be who you want to be.

Practice is Power

For me personally, I find myself on a very different wavelength from people who don't value their health. This might be in the way they eat, drink or abuse their bodies in some other way. This doesn't mean I feel superior or better than them. It just means I don't feel connected to them and their values and I won't naturally be drawn to spending a lot of time with them.

I want to spend my time with people who look after themselves and who I can have interesting, in-depth conversations with about wellbeing and living a great life, because that's what lights me up.

Coming to realisations about who you are and what you want, then figuring out whether you are surrounding yourself with people who will support you can be very confronting and uncomfortable.

But, do you know what's even more uncomfortable?

Sacrificing yourself and your ability to live your best life by wanting to please others.

That's no way to live.

Obviously, you can't change your family and you certainly don't need to give up on long-term friendships. You can, however, make an effort to nurture new relationships that support your new interests and encourage lifelong healthy habits.

Don't Preach

Food is a sensitive topic for a lot of people, and you may encounter resistance with your new choices. Instead of preaching about the virtues of the plant-based diet, the best approach is to lead by example in the way you act, look and feel. Soon enough, people will notice the change in you and ask what you're doing, at which point you can tell them and they're more likely to be receptive.

Impress your friends with a plant-based meal or encourage them to watch educational documentaries such as the ones mentioned in Chapter Six.

Most of the time, it's about how you deliver your message. People will generally respect your choices if you avoid being self-righteous or insistent.

I know of people who choose not to talk at all about their plant-based lifestyle. It's just something they 'do' while bringing as little attention to it as possible, because they don't like awkward or tricky conversations. I don't take this approach personally, but each to their own!

Celebrate Being Different

While it may be difficult to go against the grain and stand your ground, focus on all the positive aspects to your new lifestyle. A lot of people will continue to believe in their choices even when they are no longer serving them well, simply because they are entrenched and because 'it's always been that way.' As Dr Campbell notes, changes in the way society views nutrition is a paradigm shift. The more of us who participate in a plant-based lifestyle and share the benefits, the more it will become normalised. Don't be afraid to lead the way!

As with anything new, challenges will undoubtedly pop up from time to time but with practice and perseverance, soon this way of life will become your norm. Even if other people have opinions and like to share them with you, keep your resolve and know that the world around you will adjust.

Before long, people will be fascinated with your newfound glow and energy and be asking you what your secret is. You'll see!

Digging up the Dirt

Which key areas are you going to focus on first to put your new lifestyle into practice? Write down your priorities here:

_____

_____

_____

_____

_____

_____

_____

_____

_____

_____

_____

_____

_____

CHAPTER EIGHT
Effortless for Everyone

Myths and misconceptions can be a major reason why people are put off by giving the WFPB diet a try. It's a shame really, because the world would be a much better place if everyone just ate plants.

When I work with my clients and explain the benefits of this way of life – and how easy it is – they are generally very willing to jump on board and follow the guidelines, with great success. Initially, some will have concerns about how their spouse and children will adjust to the new types of meals. After a week or two, that concern generally subsides because the family members have realised that plant-based meals are actually very delicious and satisfying.

The WFPB diet is not only achievable for everybody, it is *recommended* for everybody. If you're an academic who loves research and data, I have included a list of books written by several well-respected doctors who specialise in the field of plant-based nutrition under the 'Further Reading' section at the back of the book so you can delve more deeply into the subject.

For the average adult – and particularly for the unhealthy average adult – the evidence clearly points to the advantages of a plant-based diet. But what about everyone else? Babies, toddlers, pregnant mums and athletes? Surely existing on plants must be detrimental because, shock horror, what about the protein? Sorry, that's me being facetious and making light of our society's infatuation with protein!

When you stop to think about it, doesn't it seem strange that a plant-based diet abundant in beautiful, fresh, nutrients from the earth is widely regarded as inappropriate, yet eating foods packed with artificial, man-made ingredients, sugar, gluten and fat is regarded as normal?

The purpose of this chapter is to provide an overview of what you need to know to implement the WFPB lifestyle safely during pregnancy, breastfeeding, for children and athletes. The goal is to put your mind at rest and show how easy – and healthy – it is for anyone to follow.

Much of the content in this chapter is condensed from the information obtained through my study of plant-based nutrition at Cornell University.

Pregnancy

In all honesty, I wish I had followed a plant-based diet when I was pregnant with my two kids. The whole concept just wasn't on my radar back then, and I do envy those mums-to-be who have adopted this lifestyle and are giving their children the best possible start in life. I'm not saying that not following a plant-based diet during pregnancy is bad for the mother or child, just that a plant-based diet is *better*.

Here are some of the pregnancy-related problems being created by the SAD.

Excess Protein

As we know, our society is illogically obsessed with protein intake, so a pregnant woman is likely to be given all manner of unwanted opinions on her plant-based diet by well-meaning folk who think she must be ill-informed.

It has been found that babies born to women who eat a high protein diet during pregnancy are more likely to suffer from obesity and other health issues.

In pregnancy, women retain calories, water and salt. This is becoming problematic in our modern world where so much of our everyday foods are processed and unhealthy. From an evolutionary point of view, pregnant women should actually be consuming a WFPB diet plentiful in wholegrains, legumes, soybeans, beans and lentils to get all the protein and nutrients they need. Soybeans are ideal because they contain all nine essential amino acids.

Pre-eclampsia

Pre-eclampsia is a potentially dangerous pregnancy-related condition that can lead to high blood pressure and excess protein in urine. It can cause maternal seizures, fetal growth syndrome, premature deliveries, increased c-section rates and maternal and fetal death. The condition affects roughly 5% of all pregnancies and is brought about by the body's desire to retain salt.

High blood pressure and diabetes can also cause similar issues. Medication is not a good solution because it can lead to other problems. Ideally, women should get their blood pressure and diabetes under control before falling pregnant.

A WFPB diet is ideal during pregnancy because it's typically lower in salt and reduces the risk of the above-mentioned conditions.

Macrosomia

Macrosomia is a term used to describe a much larger than average newborn. This is an escalating worldwide problem that is caused by a mother with uncontrolled diabetes, where excess sugar in the mother's system passes through to the placenta and converts into fat and creates a larger baby. Avoiding diabetes is achieved by removing high calorie, high fat foods from the diet, and therefore a low-fat, plant-based diet is ideal during pregnancy, and this should be encouraged.

Healthy Microbiome

Thankfully, the microbiome is a hot topic at the moment, so a lot of funding is being poured into research. Healthy gut microbiome has found to be important for when a baby passes through the birth canal and is exposed to the mother's bacteria, helping to build a strong immune system and protecting against future disease such as autoimmune dysfunction.

The idea that a placenta may have its own microbiome is currently being investigated to see whether an imbalance may lead to premature labour.

A plant-based diet creates healthy gut microbiome, which certainly translates to healthy fetal microbiome – another compelling reason for eating a plant-based diet during pregnancy.

Supplements

These are some supplements recommended during pregnancy:

Folic Acid: Found in leafy greens, wholegrains, legumes, fruits and vegetables and is essential for DNA repair. It helps prevent birth defects such as spina bifida and cleft palate. Those on a plant-based diet do get plenty of folic acid, but this should also be supplemented during pregnancy.

Vitamin B12: Stores can be low on a plant-based diet and this can create a risk of neural tube defects during pregnancy. Foods containing Vitamin B12 include fortified plant-based milks, cereals and nutritional yeast. A supplement should be taken every day in dropper or spray form which includes methylcobalamin as the sole ingredient.

Vitamin D: Supposed to come from sun exposure, which in turn lowers cholesterol levels. Pregnant women who live in countries where there is not much sun in the winter months (ie. Scandinavia) should take a Vitamin D supplement during pregnancy. Other sources of Vitamin D include fortified plant-based milks and sun lamps.

A Note on Iron:
There are instances when pregnant women are prescribed oral supplements, however, a word of caution here. Studies done on children and infants have shown that oral supplementation of iron can alter gut microbiome, changing it from beneficial to pathogenic. *(Pananini, D; Zimmerman, MB. Effects of iron fortification and supplementation on the gut microbiome and diarrhoea in infants and children: a review, The American Journal of Clinical Nutrition)*

This can then lead to toxic reactions with animal protein. It should also be noted that the SAD, high in calories, fat and processed food creates pathogenic microbiome. Iron supplements can cause cellular DNA damage and long-term use should be discouraged or avoided.

Pregnant women should get 27mg of iron per day and this is easily obtained on a plant-based diet, particularly through foods such as green leafy vegetables, lentils, sweet potatoes and cumin seeds.

Further plant sources of folate (folic acid) and iron include avocado, asparagus, beetroot, black beans, broccoli, figs, flaxseeds, kale, lentils, oranges, peanuts, and spinach.

A Note on DHA (Fatty Acids):
Fatty acids play an important role in brain maturation and in cell membranes, but there is little evidence to suggest supplementation is a good idea in pregnancy.

The SAD creates an imbalance of Omega 3:6 fatty acids and can interfere with enzyme activity. Vegans and those on a plant-based diet generally have normal levels of DHA. Foods such as flaxseeds contain natural essential fatty acids and should be encouraged.

Urinary Tract Infections (UTIs)

If you're female and have ever suffered the brutality of a UTI, you'll know that your doctor's plan of attack is to take a urine sample to confirm the infection, then prescribe antibiotics. There's no doubt that antibiotics kill the infection, but they also mess with your gut and can create other problems. Unfortunately – but not surprisingly – diet is not considered as a preventative treatment for UTIs, even though evidence exists that it should be.

The risk of UTIs increase on the SAD diet. When you eat meat, the acidity in an animal's intestines, along with e-coli in its gut end up colonising in your gut, leading to an increased risk of a UTI. Eliminating meat from the diet improves microbiome in the vagina and gut.

Reproductive Lifespan

The SAD is playing a significant and damaging role in terms of reproductive health and lifespan. It is creating a generation of young women in western countries who are overweight and starting menstruation earlier than in previous generations. This means the average female is experiencing more hormonal fluctuations over her lifetime and is being exposed to higher levels of oestrogen and progesterone, leading to a higher risk for breast, ovarian and uterine cancers, and a higher risk for endometriosis and fibroids.

A low fat, WFPB diet has been shown to delay the onset of menstruation for girls and decrease their risk for these health problems.

Infertility

Today, approximately 10% of couples in the west are experiencing infertility. One reason for this is many couples are delaying having children until their 30s and 40s, lowering their chances of falling pregnant. There is also a reduction in sperm count in men due to factors such as obesity and exposure to toxins from BPA, and sperm quality is being affected in men by oestrogen in dairy products.

In females, Polycystic Ovary Syndrome (PCOS) affects about 10-12% of the population and can prevent pregnancy. It's thought to sit on the same spectrum as insulin resistance (Type 2 Diabetes). As a WFPB diet is effective in treating insulin resistance, this should also be used for PCOS. Sufferers of PCOS have worse symptoms if they eat animal protein and should instead switch to plant protein.

Studies have also shown that success rates for IVF are better when the male and female follow a diet low in saturated fat, again pointing to a WFPB diet as optimal.

Interestingly, men can also experience PCOS symptoms in the form of insulin resistance which causes elevated growth factors and problems with sperm production.

Women can consume natural anti-androgens for PCOS in the form of liquorice, green tea and spearmint.

Breastfeeding

Human breastmilk contains the ideal balance of macronutrients for a baby's first year of life with 60% carbohydrate, 35% fat and 5% protein.

This raises an interesting question about why there is the belief that humans need so much protein. There is no other time in life where we grow as fast as we do in our first year, and yet 5% protein from breastmilk is adequate to support that growth.

After the natural age of weaning – historically around 2 ½ - 5 years old but much less in the modern day – humans aren't designed to continue consuming milk.

Milk Alternatives

Between the age of 0-1 year, children should be either breastfed, given human-banked milk (donor milk), or organic, non-GMO soy formula.

Whole cow's milk should not be given to infants under one year of age because it is poorly digested by an immature gut and is linked to atopic (allergic) and autoimmune sickness. The composition of cow's milk differs a lot from human milk because it contains up to 27% protein. Cheese and yoghurt are also a problem because they contain casein and are inflammatory in the body.

Soy formula products do have sugars, but they are the best available alternative to breast milk. They are *not* suitable for premature babies or for babies diagnosed with a milk protein or soy allergy. Babies in this category should be given a hydrolysed cow's milk formula, which is where the cow's milk proteins have been broken down by enzymes into very small particles called peptides.

Goat's milk is very similar to cow's milk and is not recommended for children, nor is raw milk from any animal due to the risk of bacterial contamination.

Between the ages of 1-2 years, children should either be breastfed, or if they are weaning and have good growth and good eating patterns, it's fine to wean them onto water. If the child has poor growth and is a fussy eater, fortified, organic, unsweetened soy milk containing healthy fats and proteins is recommended. If the child already eats soy products, hemp milk is recommended instead.

For an older child who needs to restrict calories, almond milk is an ideal option. Coconut milk is not recommended due to high quantities of saturated fat, and rice milk should be limited due to possible arsenic contamination. Be sure to check the nutritional labels on milk cartons and choose one that has been minimally processed without added oils and sweeteners.

Humans are the only species to drink the milk of another species after weaning. Dairy products are not necessary in a child's diet and all beneficial components of dairy products can be found elsewhere.

Butter is 100% fat, cheese is 75% fat and milk is 50% fat and is the number one source of saturated fat in the human diet. The staggering fat content in cow's milk is designed to grow a calf into a cow, not to optimise health in humans.

Here are some other quick facts relating to dairy products and their detrimental effect on human health:

- Casein found in milk is a potent carcinogen.
- 75% of people around the world are lactose intolerant.
- High levels of oestrogen and progesterone in milk contributes to issues such as acne, breast cancer, PCOS and early puberty.
- High levels of insulin growth factor (IGF – 1) in cows (resulting from the injection of growth hormones to

stimulate milk production) promote the growth of cancer cells.
- All animal products have highly concentrated levels of pesticides and other environmental contaminants.
- There are increasing problems related to antibiotic-resistant strains of bacteria due to the quantities of antibiotics given to dairy cattle.
- Dairy proteins can stimulate immunological reactions when absorbed through inflamed intestinal lining, also known as 'gut leakage'.

Solids for Babies

Taste preferences at the age of 20 are generally established by age two. It goes without saying that a child who is never introduced to foods such as meat, eggs and dairy products will not develop the taste for them.

Babies are ready to try new tastes between the age of four and seven months. Good WFPB options include wholegrain cereals, fruits, green vegetables and legumes. Babies who are exposed to allergenic foods (such as peanuts) during this time have shown to be at less risk of allergic reactions as they get older. Whole nuts are actually a choking hazard and shouldn't be given to children until 3-4 years old, so nut butters are a better option.

High intake of animal protein at a young age has shown to lead to early menstruation for girls, and as already discussed, this can cause problems later in life, particularly related to cancer development.

Nutrition for Children

Chronic disease that develops in adulthood generally begin in childhood, although it can be decades before symptoms appear.

According to research done by Dr Michael Greger, the following applies to the SAD:

- By age 10, 100% of children have fatty streaks in their arteries.
- By early 20s, 77% have fully formed plaque, some with vessels up to 90% occluded.
- By 30s and 40s, plaque progresses.
- By 50s and 60s, there are outward symptoms of heart disease.

The following factors contribute to excess cancer rates in children, particularly reproductive cancers such as breast, ovarian and prostate:

- Less fruit consumption
- More meat consumption
- Being overweight in childhood
- Higher overall calorie consumption in childhood
- Earlier puberty
- Rapid growth at an early age.

Type 2 Diabetes is being seen in children as young as eight years old and is strongly correlated with childhood obesity. A scary fact is that even if an overweight child loses weight later in life, the risks associated with childhood obesity remain.

Other health issues associated with the SAD in children include asthma, eczema, allergies, ADHD and acne.

The earlier a child starts to follow a WFPB diet, the greater the benefits to overall health, and the reduced risk for cancer, obesity, heart disease, diabetes and other chronic illness.

Between the ages of birth to three years, there is a higher requirement for fat, protein and calorie density in the diet. From three years onward, there are no special dietary requirements.

For children aged 3+ their protein needs range between 7-14% of overall calories, whereas the average intake on the SAD is 15-25%.

Children have high energy needs in childhood and need calorie-dense, nutrient-dense foods at every meal such as nuts, seeds, starchy vegetables, avocados, legumes, wholegrains, and beans.

Development and Growth

Children on a WFPB diet have been shown to have a longer duration for growth, later and sometimes slower growth spurts, and equal to greater height compared to those on the SAD. The onset of puberty typically starts later, with girls beginning menstruation later.

Soy products are often touted as troublesome but in fact are shown to be beneficial to the reproductive system. Good sources of soy include soy milk, tofu, tempeh and soybeans. Intake of soy in childhood has been found to be more protective to health compared with intake in adulthood.

There is no greater risk for eating disorders in children who follow a WFPB diet. A sensible, healthy approach to food is to focus on the abundance of food types available and to promote a relaxed enjoyment around food.

Your doctor may express some concern when you inform them your child is following a WFPB diet because as we know, the SAD is considered 'normal'. How sad is that? You can be respectful towards their beliefs while being confident in yours at the same time. Any doctor worth their salt will support you in your decisions and help you ensure your chid is healthy.

With children who are fussy eaters, unfortunately there is no magic bullet. My kids have been around a WFPB diet for a few years now, and they still screw their noses up at their meals more often than I would like. I have found that the more times they are exposed to a certain type of food, the more they come to accept that it's just part of life, and over time, they will eat it without question.

Don't expect miracles overnight, but do be careful not to offer too many alternative options or get sucked into having to cook separate meals for your kids. If they have a choice between a chickpea curry and a cheesy lasagne, they will most likely choose the lasagne every time – let's be honest! However, if the lasagne isn't available to start with, they will be left with no other option than to eat the healthier plant-based option.

When it comes to kids, practice, patience and perseverance is key.

Macronutrients

These are some great plant-based carbohydrate, protein and fat options for children:

Whole food, plant-based carbohydrate options:
- All vegetables (potatoes, sweet potatoes, kumara, pumpkin are great)

- Brown rice
- Whole wheat pasta (preferably gluten free)
- Whole grain or sprouted bread (preferably gluten free)
- Quinoa
- Oats
- Buckwheat
- All fruits including berries
- Kidney beans
- Chickpeas

Whole food, plant-based protein options:
- Lentils
- Chickpeas
- Peanuts
- Almonds
- Spirulina
- Quinoa*
- Soybeans*
- Tofu, tempeh, edamame
- Chia seeds
- Hemp seeds
- Beans with rice*
- Potatoes
- Green leafy vegetables

*These are complete proteins, meaning they contain adequate proportions of each of the nine essential amino acids.

Whole food, plant-based fat options:
- Avocado
- Flaxseed
- Hemp seeds
- Olive oil

- Peanuts
- Tahini
- Nuts and seeds
- Chia seeds
- Cacao nibs
- Coconut

Essential Fatty Acids (EFAs):
The information pertaining to EFAs on page 66 also applies to children.

Micronutrients

These are some key points around micronutrients (vitamins and minerals) as they specifically relate to children:

Calcium
- Casein in dairy products is a potent carcinogen (cancer causing).
- All beneficial components of milk can be found elsewhere.
- Plant-based forms of calcium are better absorbed than dairy products.

Whole-food, plant-based calcium options:
- Green leafy veggies such as broccoli, kale, cabbage, okra and bok choy
- Fortified unsweetened soy, rice and oat milks
- Tofu
- Sesame seeds
- Tahini
- Pulses
- Dried fruit such as raisins, prunes, figs and dried apricots

- Orange juice
- Chia seeds and hemp seeds
- Oats
- Berries such as blackberries and raspberries
- Beans such as kidney beans

Vitamin D

The information pertaining to Vitamin D on page 73 also applies to children.

Iron
- Heme iron (animal origin) is readily absorbed, difficult to regulate and there is a risk of overload.
- Absorption of non-heme iron (vegetable origin) is easily regulated and there is no risk of overload.
- Plant-based children get more iron from their food than meat eaters.
- Iron-rich foods should ideally be paired with Vitamin C-rich foods for better absorption.

Whole-food, plant-based options for iron:
- Lentils
- Chickpeas
- Beans
- Tofu
- Cashew nuts
- Chia seeds
- Ground linseed
- Hemp seeds
- Pumpkin seeds
- Kale
- Dried apricots and figs
- Raisins

- Quinoa
- Fortified breakfast cereal
- Spirulina

Taking oral supplements can alter gut bacteria (as shown by studies conducted in children), and chronic consumption should be avoided because it can cause cellular damage. It's reasonable to include a child's multivitamin if kids are picky eaters or if there are any other concerns.

Bone Health

Data linking bone health to calcium is insufficient, and in fact the countries with the highest calcium intake from dairy products also have the highest rates of osteoporosis. *(Lanau, A; PhD, Nutrition Director for the Physicians Committee for Responsible Medicine, Washington DC)*

More importantly than calcium intake, good bone health is achieved by adequate exposure to Vitamin D (sunshine), a low sodium diet, weight bearing exercise, avoiding excess dietary protein (especially animal) and an alkaline diet high in fruits and vegetables. For strong bones, children should get about three hours of exercise every day.

Supplementation for Children

Here's a list of supplements recommended for children following a WFPB diet:

Vitamin B12
The information pertaining to Vitamin B12 on page 72 also applies to children. Specific doses for children are as follows:

Vitamin B12 Requirements by Age:

4-13 years	1.2mcg per day
14+ years	2.5mcg per day

Babies should be given Vitamin B12 once they are no longer receiving large amounts of calories from breast milk. If the mother is low in B12, babies should be supplemented straight away in gummy or spray form. Appropriate dosages are given below.

0-12 months	0.5mcg per day
1-3 years	1mcg per day

Liquid Zinc Sulphate
Another potent workhorse, liquid zinc sulphate is anti-viral and is responsible for good liver function, skin and wound healing, sexual function, insulin and growth hormones.

Spirulina
Responsible for detoxing toxic heavy metals from the body, liver detox, prevents viral and bacterial growth inside the liver and iron deficiency.

Barley Grass Powder
Great for toxic heavy metal detox, stomach issues, feeds the liver and is a potent detoxifier.

Lypospheric Vitamin C
Excellent to have on hand for immunity and to assist with iron absorption.

I recommend all five supplements noted above to most age groups for optimal health. Please make sure you read the nutritional label for correct dosages according to age, and if unsure, speak to your pharmacist.

Extra Snack Ideas for Kids

Ideally, keep snacks dairy and gluten free where possible:

- Whole fruit
- Dried fruit
- Veggie sticks and hummus
- Sushi
- Mini muffins
- Bliss balls
- Nuts and raisins
- Mini pancakes/pikelets
- Tofu cubes
- Pizza
- Crackers
- Plain potato chips
- Popcorn
- Banana bread
- Falafel
- Fruit gummies
- Mini chocolate mousse
- Rice cakes / corn thins with peanut butter and banana/avocado etc.
- Fruit skewers
- Smoothies – so many options but always good to include spirulina/barley grass.
- Use any of my sweet recipes on my Facebook page for a healthy treat.

Nutrition for Athletes

If you google 'plant-based athletes', you will come across many elite athletes who are turning to a WFPB in an effort to gain an edge over their competitors, with spectacular results. World Number 1 tennis player, Novak Djokovic, credits a WFPB diet for his rise from third in the world to first.

> "My performance has improved since I have eaten plant-based. I think that's one of the reasons I recover well. I don't have any allergies that I used to have any more."
>
> (Novak Djokovic)

Champion Formula One driver, Lewis Hamilton, has said that his change to a WFPB diet made all the difference in his career, and ultra-marathon runner, Scott Jurek, winner of 16 ultramarathon titles, has claimed his vegan diet is crucial in supporting his endurance, recovery and overall health.

The general consensus from WFPB athletes is that they achieve superior performance, better recovery, increased energy levels and become bigger and stronger without the use of supplementation.

Recovery is a key consideration for athletes, because exercise creates inflammation in the body. WFPB foods are anti-inflammatory, particularly things like ginger and turmeric. Any athlete eating this way is going to have superior recovery over an athlete on the SAD.

The following information relating to nutrition for athletes is obtained from a combination of my husband Steve's background in performance nutrition, research from plant-based doctors such as Dr Neal Barnard, and information taught by Cornell University.

Protein

Contrary to popular belief, high quantities of protein do not equate to better athletic performance. Below are some key points to note when it comes to this macronutrient:

- Too much protein puts excess stress on the kidneys, liver and bones.
- Studies have shown that decreasing protein intake to 64g per day can increase performance by 35%. *(Chittenden, R H. (1904). Physiological economy in nutrition, with special reference to the minimal protein requirement of the healthy man. An experimental study. New York: Frederick A. Stokes Company)*
- Adults can't increase muscle mass by eating excessive amounts of protein. Muscle is determined by genetics, hormones, and the frequency of muscle loading (weightlifting).
- Too much protein is harmful because it leads to insufficient carbohydrate stores to replenish muscle glycogen. This can cause dehydration and fluid imbalances.
- Athletes only need 10% of their calories from protein to put their bodies into positive nitrogen balance. Ideally, the goal is to reach positive nitrogen balance and stay there, not exceed it. Nitrogen balance is a measure of nitrogen intake minus nitrogen loss. Plant-based sources of nitrogen intake include grains, nuts, legumes, and cereals. Nitrogen losses include urine, faeces, sweat, hair and skin.
- Caloric needs determine how much food is required and is regulated by the brain and hunger signals (see Harris Benedict Formula on page 160).
- Each main meal should ideally have a wholegrain, a protein such as legumes, tofu or beans, plus vegetables.

Endurance Athletes

The diet of an endurance athlete should be based on calorie-dense complex carbohydrates, low in fat and abundant in vitamins, minerals and antioxidants to support performance. Ideal foods include potatoes, beans, lentils, squash, brown rice, oats, quinoa, and fruit – especially before workouts.

The release of free radicals during intense exercise causes cell damage, loss of muscle function and an inflammatory response in the body. The nutrition provided by a WFPB diet assists in short and long-term recovery.

Pre-Workout

Here are some pre-workout food guidelines for elite athletes:

Carbohydrate : Protein ratio 3:1

Focus on dates, pineapple, apricots, cherries, which are high in glucose, and nuts for protein.

One hour before the workout, choose from:

- Apples
- Bananas
- Nut butter

For example, almond butter on apple slices.

Two hours before the workout, choose from:

- Porridge, nuts and ground flaxseed will achieve the 3:1 ratio
- Wholegrain bread or toast with peanut butter and jam
- Muesli with plant-based milk

Fuel with carbohydrates before and during exercise to prevent glucose depletion.

During Workout

A good guideline is to consume 120-240 calories per hour or 30-60g of carbohydrates per hour during exercise.

You can exercise for approximately two hours (on average) before running out of glycogen, depending on the intensity of the exercise and individual needs.

Good sources of fuel during a longer workout include:

- Bananas
- Watermelons
- Raisins
- Mashed potato (mash and put into bags, bite off corner and squeeze)

Post-Workout

Immediately after exercise: replenish glycogen with a 3:1 or 4:1 ratio of carbohydrates to protein. Focus on bananas, nuts and seeds.

45-60 minute after exercise: focus on plant-based protein such as legumes, quinoa and leafy greens.

1-2 hours after exercise: focus on pasta, vegetables, and lentils.

Other important considerations after exercise include foam rolling, stretching, massage and compression socks. Good options if you require extra snacks include fruit, green smoothies, nuts and dried fruit.

Hydration

Adequate hydration is essential before, during and after exercise to ensure optimal performance, but be sure to avoid over-drinking. If you are in the lead up to a big event, drink an extra one or two cups of water per day on top of what you normally would. Urine should run clear if you are well hydrated. During exercise, consume 120-180ml of water every 10-20 minutes. The aim is to replace what you lose in body weight.

'Sports drinks' such as *Powerade* or *Gatorade* are full of sugar and other unnecessary ingredients, and it is best to make your own sports drink at home — there are plenty of resources available online to show you how. Coconut water is very hydrating and high in electrolytes.

High-quality anti-inflammatory foods to assist with recovery include turmeric and ginger, green leafy vegetables, nuts and fruit.

Add a pea protein powder into smoothies if you feel you need the extra calories and feeling of being full.

Full o' Beans!

The Harris Benedict Formula

The Harris Benedict Formula calculates how many calories are needed per day. Multiply your Basal Metabolic Rate (BMR) by your physical activity factor. (BMR = how many calories your body needs just to survive).

Men:
BMR = (10 x weight in kg) + (6.25 x height in cm) − (5 x age in years) + 5

Women:
BMR = (10 x weight in kg) + (6.25 x height in cm) − (5 x age in years) -161.

Once you have the BMR, multiply by your level of activity, as follows:

Sedentary	BMR x 1.2	(little or no exercise)
Lightly active	BMR x 1.375	(light exercise 1-3 days per week)
Moderately active	BMR x 1.55	(exercise 3-5 days per week)
Very active	BMR x 1.725	(exercise 6-7 days per week)
Extremely active	BMR x 1.9	(hard training / physical job)

This calculation will provide your total number of required calories per day.

The information presented in this chapter clearly shows the benefits for all who follow a WFPB diet. I don't know about you, but the thing that bothers me the most about the SAD is what's happening with our children. While under their parent or guardian's roof, children have very little say or control about what they eat. By the time they are independent, their conditioning and habits are ingrained and very difficult to change. That's why an overweight child is very likely to become an overweight adult and stay that way for life.

As adults, we absolutely must do better for our kids. A perfect diet is unrealistic, but the rates of chronic childhood illnesses show that we must take control of the situation and stop killing our young people prematurely. Talking or reading about the issue isn't good enough – it's our job to lead by example and show our kids how to lead a healthy and balanced lifestyle.

How do we do that? By our own actions, of course.

Yet again, I encourage you to take a good look around you for all the blatant evidence you need that our current SAD state of affairs just isn't working. Podgy bellies, sky-high blood pressure and chronic disease are no longer the domain of retired old men. Much of our population, starting from a very young age, now have something wrong with their health.

It's such a big problem that it's tempting to throw it in the too-hard basket. If you're thinking, *"But, what can I do about it?"*, the first place to start is with ourselves, and our own families. Commit to doing things differently from now on and follow through with your actions.

It's not easy, but it's definitely worth it – and your impact is bigger than you realise. Don't underestimate the power of the ripple effect and the positive influence you can have on the world around you.

Digging up the Dirt

How do your lifestyle choices affect those around you? What are the things you'd like to commit to doing differently from now on?

_____
_____
_____
_____
_____
_____
_____
_____
_____
_____
_____
_____

CHAPTER NINE
Healthy and Happy

Kylie's Story

In September 2018, I was diagnosed with urticaria (chronic hives) by a doctor and skin specialist. I was prescribed antihistamine to help with the itch and was told the condition could last up to six months. Over two years later, at the beginning of 2021, it was still driving me crazy, so I went back to the doctor for more tests. Nothing unusual showed up and I was prescribed more antihistamine. I was also prescribed anti-depressants but didn't take them. I was feeling low, but knew I wasn't depressed.

I decided to go and see Heidi to see if she could help me, and we discussed everything I was going through. Thinking back to that first meeting, I was completely stressed out, juggling work, family life and this annoying urticaria. Heidi gave me an adrenal stress quiz to complete, and my score was quite high, revealing my body was not in a good state. My quality of life was suffering, and I needed some help.

Heidi suggested I start on her plant-based holistic coaching programme, which included easy-to-follow meal plans and regular zoom coaching sessions to keep me on track. Through the programme, I eliminated some troublesome foods and learned which foods would trigger my skin and cause me to itch. The itching reduced significantly in just a few weeks, and I was able to start reducing my medication. Originally, my doctor had put me on two antihistamine tablets each day.

Completing Heidi's programme was a great experience for me. She is very helpful and really knows her stuff. I enjoyed the weekly coaching sessions, which kept me accountable and gave me the opportunity to ask questions and make sure I was progressing. The meal plans were super easy to follow, and the food tasted great, with plenty of variety. As an added bonus, I lost a few kilos, too!

Today, by continuing to follow the guidelines Heidi taught me, I take only one or two antihistamine tablets each month, and no longer have any major skin flare ups. Not having to rely on medication anymore means my quality of life has improved and I don't have to worry about the consequences of what will happen to my skin if I accidentally miss taking the tablets.

I would recommend Heidi's programme to anyone suffering from health issues that are affecting their quality of life. Changing your diet can make all the difference.

Kylie Teague, 44

Jenny's Story

When I first came to see Heidi, I was not in great condition. I was drinking too much coffee to get me through the day, then beer at night to wind down. My sleep was poor, I had hot sweats, cramps, recurring eczema and brain fog which made work difficult.

I was really struggling to address minor problems in life; everything was so hard. I had no energy and didn't want to get out of bed in the morning. I was feeling anxious and very overwhelmed.

I found the first two weeks on the coaching programme the hardest, but I knew I had to make changes, so I stuck with it. I cut down my coffee intake to one per day and started cutting back on alcohol. These changes made a huge difference.

I enjoyed the meal plans because they gave me structure during the week, and it was helpful having the grocery list all ready to go. My partner is a meat eater but the meal plan was good because it was flexible and allowed for him to eat meat.

The programme made such a huge difference to me. After just a few weeks, I had lots of energy. I had heard people say they bounce out of bed in the morning, and I thought, yeah right! But it started happening for me, too! I was coping with everything much better and enjoying my life.

I feel 200% better now. Walking has become easier and now I walk every morning. I am enjoying work again and getting stuck into my garden. I enjoy cooking and searching for new recipes. My enthusiasm is now 10-fold to what it was. I am so much happier.

I am so grateful to have had Heidi's assistance throughout the programme. It kept me accountable, and it was good to have that help on hand when things got a bit tough. I spoke to Heidi every week for the first four weeks, then we stretched our remaining coaching sessions out to fortnightly. That was great because it was empowering for me to know I could deal with things on my own. I knew I could call or email Heidi for help if I needed it. That was worth gold.

I would recommend this programme to anyone and everyone, because it actually works!

Jenny, 66

Nola's Story

When I first went to see Heidi, I was a complete mess and hanging by a thread. I was in so much pain and so tired and didn't know what to do. I had fibromyalgia, asthma, diverticulitis, chronic pain and anxiety. My problems were affecting me deeply. I was trying to do the housework, cook the meals, play bowls when I could, play bridge, go to aqua aerobics and book club and look after the grandchildren in the school holidays. I was eating comfort food like chocolate, biscuits and potato chips and wasn't sleeping. I put on a brave face, but my body wasn't happy.

I had seen what Heidi had been through with her own health transformation so thought I could really learn something from her. I had to trust someone who was going to show me how to eat properly and listen to my body. Heidi was instantly loving and kind and I was able to tell her how I was feeling. I think the best possible advice she gave me was to STOP doing all the things I thought I should be doing and rest.

Through the coaching programme, I could call Heidi at any time and ask her questions. I realised very quickly how good the programme was and found I started to feel a lot better very quickly. My judgement was getting better, and I certainly didn't have as much pain.

My first thought when I saw the food plan was, "I can't do that!", but I had made a commitment to myself so gave it a go. I found I liked a lot of the meals and snacks, and they were very satisfying. Now I love the food and my cooking has improved so much! I also know I can go out to a café or restaurant and make good choices. Weight loss wasn't a priority, but I lost 7kg which was great for me. I watch the scales now and am happier and more confident.

I am now dairy and gluten-free and it's so much better for me. I do like the 80/20 rule though – it's liberating as I can have my 'cheats' and not feel guilty.

After a few weeks, my health was so much better. I had more energy, strength, mental capacity and was more organised. My asthma and anxiety had improved, and the pain from the diverticulitis and fibromyalgia was diminishing. Because of the COVID—19 pandemic situation, I was enjoying getting some rest. I started to think of others more than myself and made sure I called on friends and family more often. I now listen to my body and don't feel guilty when I need a rest during the day.

My quality of life improved so much. For three years beforehand, I kept telling my husband I wanted to move into a retirement village so I could go to the hospital there and be looked after. Well, that hasn't happened! We have now done a little renovation on our house with new carpet and paint. If you had told me a few months ago that I would be decluttering my home of 32 years, I would have said you were nuts. But, I've done it!

I would recommend this programme to everyone because it is life changing.

Nola Darvill, 77

CHAPTER TEN
Delectable Dining

We are now at the part of the book where you can get your hands dirty – or keep them clean, depending on what type of cook you are!

There's been a lot to learn about the plant-based lifestyle in the previous chapters, and I know it can seem somewhat daunting in the beginning. But trust me when I say it's so much easier than you may think, especially when you have someone guiding you through the process.

In this chapter, I am going to share with you everything you need to know about making a start with this new and exciting way of life.

Remember, changing the way you eat doesn't have to be swift and dramatic. Factors such as your current lifestyle, workload, budget, and family circumstances will dictate the types of changes you decide to make, and when.

The whole idea behind this lifestyle is to get you feeling great, so creating more stress is not what this is all about! If small, gradual changes work best for you, that is absolutely fine. Or maybe you're a sweeping-change-all-at-once type of person, and that's fine, too. Do what feels right for you.

We are going to discuss how to stock your kitchen to ensure great success with this new way of life, and I'm also going to share some of my favourite, tried and tested recipes for you to try.

Stocking Your Kitchen

Cooking healthy, plant-based meals is so much more enjoyable when you have the right ingredients on hand. There's nothing worse than getting excited about trying a new recipe, then realising you're not prepared.

If re-stocking your kitchen all at once doesn't fit your budget, you can start by swapping items one at a time with a healthier option each time you go shopping. Most plant-based grocery items are actually fairly basic and cost-effective and can be used in all sorts of different ways.

With bulk items, dry goods and produce, I recommend buying organic and local ingredients as often as possible, but just do the best you can.

The key thing I recommend you do in the beginning is get rid of all the processed junk foods in your fridge and pantry, such as bags of chips, cookies, snack foods loaded with white sugar and flour and sugar-filled spreads. By doing this, you are literally wiping the slate clean and making way for healthy options, which will give you a real psychological boost and give you the best chance of success.

Here are some staples for a plant-based pantry and fridge, many of which will be used in the recipes to follow later in the chapter. Please note that not all of these ingredients are essential or need to be bought all at once, and whether you buy them will depend on personal preference.

Dried Goods:
- Whole wheat pasta
- Brown rice
- Basmati rice
- Black rice
- Dried chickpeas
- Dried black beans
- Dried kidney beans
- Canned chickpeas
- Canned black beans
- Canned lentils
- Canned diced tomatoes
- Orange, green, red lentils
- Quinoa
- Unsweetened coconut milk
- Extra virgin olive oil
- Organic coconut oil
- All-purpose gluten-free flour
- Apple cider vinegar
- Nutritional yeast

Full o' Beans!

Nuts, Seeds, Dried Fruits:
- Walnuts
- Almonds
- Pecans
- Cashews
- Flaxseeds
- Chia seeds
- Sunflower seeds
- Pumpkin seeds
- Dried mango
- Dried pineapple
- Dried ginger
- Dried banana
- Banana chips
- Coconut

Dried Spices:
- Allspice
- Basil
- Bay leaves
- Black peppercorns
- Cayenne pepper
- Chilli powder / flakes
- Cinnamon
- Cloves
- Coriander
- Cumin
- Curry powder
- Dill

- Garam masala
- Garlic powder
- Nutmeg
- Onion powder
- Oregano
- Paprika
- Powdered ginger
- Rosemary
- Sage
- Tarragon
- Thyme
- Turmeric

Plant-Based Chocolate:
When buying plant-based chocolate, read labels carefully and avoid artificial flavourings and food starch. Plant-based chocolate doesn't include dairy products and you will want a high-quality, dark variety which is made with natural ingredients such as cacao, cacao butter, limited sugar and vanilla. I personally like the *Lindt* brand (85% or 90%).

- Cacao nibs
- Chocolate-covered almonds
- Cacao powder
- Dark chocolate
- Chocolate spread

Sweet Toppings/Recipe add-ins:
- Brown rice syrup
- Caramel sauce
- Peanut butter
- Coconut sugar
- Chocolate sauce
- Maple syrup

Optional for Smoothies:
- Plant protein powder
- Spirulina
- Barley grass powder
- Acai powder
- Rolled oats
- Algae
- Beet powder
- Turmeric
- Flaxseed

Freezer:
Variety of frozen fruits for smoothies and smoothie bowls, such as:
- Ripe bananas
- Mangos (cut into chunks)
- Pineapple (cut into chunks)
- Blueberries
- Acai packets
- Pitaya (dragon fruit)
- Strawberries
- Soups

- Avocados about to go off to be used in smoothies/chocolate mousse

Fridge:
Vegetables:
- Spinach
- Kale
- Cucumbers
- Carrots
- Potatoes
- Sweet potatoes
- Broccoli
- Cauliflower
- Purple cabbage
- Green cabbage
- Tomatoes
- Red onions
- White or yellow onions
- Garlic

Fresh Herbs:
- Chives
- Coriander
- Mint
- Parsley
- Basil
- Rosemary

Condiments:
- Capers
- Olives
- Pickled red onions
- Homemade sauces
- Mustard
- Teriyaki sauce
- Coconut aminos / Tamari sauce
- Worcestershire sauce (vegan)
- Pickled ginger
- Miso paste
- Red curry paste

Plant Milks:
Aim for a plant milk that is unsweetened and organic.
- Almond milk
- Oat milk
- Rice milk
- Soy milk
- Hemp milk

Fruits:
Choose your favourite fruits that are in season for snacks or to add to smoothie bowls, such as:
- Apples
- Bananas
- Kiwis
- Grapes
- Pears

Delectable Dining

- Berries
- Papaya
- Mango
- Pineapple

Other
- Sourdough bread (preferably gluten-free)
- Corn tortillas
- Corn chips
- Pita bread (gluten-free)
- Tofu

Recipes

Now for the super fun part... The recipes! There are an infinite number of plant-based recipes available now on the internet, in cookbooks, YouTube etc, and sharing all my favourites would take another whole book! For now, here are just a few of my tried and tested winners that are relatively simple and will give you a good introduction to plant-based eating and how delicious and easy it can be:

JUICES AND SMOOTHIES

Chunky Chai Milkshake

This shake is packed with nutrients with a chocolate-chai flavour. You can adjust spice quantities to suit your taste.

- 1 ½ cups plant milk of choice (rice/oat/soy/almond)
- 1 frozen ripe banana
- 1 tbsp cacao powder
- 1/2 tsp ground cinnamon
- 1/8 tsp ground nutmeg
- 1/8 tsp ground cloves
- 1/8 tsp ground cardamom
- 1/4 tsp ground ginger
- 1/2 tsp vanilla extract
- 1 piece crystalised ginger or 1 tsp grated ginger (optional)
- Pitted dates (Medjool are ideal) or 1 tbsp maple syrup
- 1 cup ice

1. Place all ingredients in a high-speed blender.
2. Blend on medium speed, then on high for 1-2 minutes or until the milkshake is creamy and smooth. You may need to stop the blender a few times to mix the ingredients together and push them down with a tamper or smoothie stick.

Heidi's Green Monster Smoothie

My Green Monster smoothie definitely deserves its moment of fame! I regularly give this to my clients for overall sparkling health and wellbeing. It's particularly great for sharp mental focus and clearing brain fog.

Makes 1 large serving or more if you add extra liquid.

- 1 banana
- 1 handful frozen fruit of choice (mango is great)
- 1 large handful fresh spinach
- 1-2 tsp spirulina
- 1-2 tsp barley grass powder
- 1 cup coconut water
- Splash of plant-based milk of choice (coconut milk makes it creamy)
- Extra water to bulk up if you like

1. Blend all ingredients together.
2. Serve in a tall glass.
3. Go back for seconds – it's that good!

Spring Breeze Juice

Imagine a hot day, lounging beneath a palm tree on your favourite beach with a gentle breeze caressing your skin. If you could choose the perfect drink to be placed in your hand, it would have to be this one. Aptly named the 'Spring Breeze' because of its refreshing, zesty taste, this juice will make your insides sing!

Serves 2

- 4 green apples, cored and quartered
- 2 whole cucumbers, roughly chopped
- 5-6 stalks celery, roughly chopped
- Leaves of 4 mint sprigs
- Juice of 1 lime

1. Place all ingredients into a juicer and juice.
2. Serve in a tall glass with ice.

NB: Make sure you use a juicer, not a blender – they are two very different appliances!

BREAKFAST

Chocolate Berry Overnight Oats

This is a delicious, super-filling breakfast option which only takes a couple of minutes to prepare the night before. Who said you can't have chocolate for breakfast?

Serves 2

- 1 cup unsweetened non-dairy milk (rice/oat/soy/almond/hemp)
- 2-3 pitted dates
- 1 tbsp raisins
- 1 large banana
- 1 tbsp cacao or cocoa powder
- 1 cup rolled oats
- 1 cup frozen or fresh berries

1. Blend the milk with the dates, raisins, banana and cacao or cocoa.
2. Combine blended milk with oats in a medium bowl.
3. Add berries and stir well.
4. Cover and refrigerate for at least 1 hour or overnight.
5. If you prefer, you can warm the oats up in the microwave the next morning, or eat cold.

Scrambled Tofu

Scrambled eggs on toast is one of those comfort foods that you just can't beat, except of course if you're plant-based! Tofu scramble is a great plant-based alternative, providing a similar taste and texture, but without the eggs.

This recipe is super quick and easy and so tasty you will want to go back for more!

Serves 2

- 2 tbsp vegetable oil
- 1 large onion, diced
- 2 tsp garlic, crushed

- 2 tomatoes, diced
- 1 block tofu, crumbled
- 1 tsp turmeric
- 1 tsp paprika
- ½ tsp nutritional yeast (optional)
- 1 tsp sea salt, or to taste
- Black pepper, to taste
- Pinch cayenne pepper
- 1 tbsp soy sauce or tamari sauce, or to taste

1. Put oil in a large skillet on medium-high heat. Add onion and garlic and cook until onions are soft and translucent, approximately 5 minutes. Stir frequently.
2. Add tofu and cook for 5 minutes, stirring occasionally. Add remaining ingredients and cook for another 5 minutes, stirring occasionally.
3. Serve on warm toast or with a side of veggie sausages or hash browns.

Banana and Strawberry Pancakes

You can't go wrong with a stack of pancakes for Sunday brunch. And unlike the regular gluten and sugar-heavy variety, these ones won't leave you feeling sluggish and in need of a nap! These pancakes are a great way to fuel a busy day ahead.

Serves 4

- 1 ripe banana, mashed
- 1 cup gluten free flour
- 1 tsp baking powder
- ½ tsp baking soda

- 1 tsp lemon juice
- ¾ cup almond milk
- ¾ cup strawberries, sliced (can use frozen and thawed)
- 2 tbsp coconut oil
- 2 tbsp coconut yoghurt
- 2 tbsp maple syrup

1. Mash the bananas with a fork and combine them with the flour, baking powder, baking soda and lemon juice. Next, slowly add in almond milk until you get a thick batter.
2. Finally, fold in the sliced strawberries, leaving some for garnish.
3. Heat some of the oil in a non-stick pan over medium heat, not too hot to burn the pancakes.
4. Spoon a little less than ¼ cup of the batter per pancake (this will make around 8 pancakes).
5. Cook for about 3 minutes on one side, then when bubbles start to appear flip and cook for another minute.
6. Serve the pancakes with a tablespoon of coconut yoghurt and maple syrup, and garnish with remaining strawberries.

LUNCH

Mexican Black Bean Bowl

This Mexican-inspired dish is so tasty and full of nutrients that it will keep you well fuelled for hours.

Serves 2

- 2 tbsp extra virgin olive oil
- 1 large sweet potato

Full o' Beans!

- ½ tsp paprika
- Salt & freshly ground black pepper
- 1 can black beans, drained and rinsed (or other legumes such as lentils / chickpeas)
- ¼ tsp chilli powder
- ½ tsp garlic powder
- Juice of 2-3 limes, plus 1 tbsp lime juice
- 2 medium tomatoes, diced
- ½ cup diced white onion
- ½ cup finely chopped coriander leaves
- ½ cup corn kernels
- 1 cup shredded romaine lettuce

Toppings: coriander leaves, diced avocado, tortilla strips, lime wedges

1. Preheat the oven to 220 degrees Celsius.
2. Cut the sweet potato into 2cm cubes. Place in a medium bowl, toss with olive oil and paprika, and season with salt and pepper. Roast for 40 minutes or until slightly browned.
3. Put the black beans in a small saucepan. Place over medium heat and mix in the chilli powder and garlic powder. Cook for 3-5 minutes, until the black beans are warm. Stir in the 1 tbsp of lime juice.
4. Combine the tomatoes, onion, the juice of 2 limes, and the coriander in a small bowl. Taste and add the juice of the third lime if needed. Set aside.
5. To build your bowls, divide the black beans, roasted sweet potatoes, corn, lettuce and tomato mixture between bowls. Add any of the suggested toppings. Drizzle with your favourite dairy-free dressing and serve.

Recipes

Lentil and Pumpkin Soup

You can't beat a bowl of warm, delicious soup. This one has a rich, creamy texture and tastes amazing!

Makes 8 x 1 cup serves

- 1 ½ cups onion, diced
- 2 stalks celery, diced
- 1 tbsp chopped ginger or puree
- 1 tbsp oil
- 1 tsp turmeric
- 2 tsp mild curry powder
- 5 cups boiling water
- 1 cup red lentils
- 3 cups chopped pumpkin
- 1 ½ tsp salt
- 200ml coconut cream / milk
- Juice of 2 limes

Garnish: Parsley

1. Sauté onion, celery, ginger and oil in a large soup pot until onion is clear.
2. Add spices and mix for about 30 seconds.
3. Add water, lentils and pumpkin and simmer for approximately 15 minutes or until the lentils are soft and pumpkin is cooked.
4. Place the mixture in a high-powered blender and blend until smooth (you may need to do this in several batches depending on the size of your blender).
5. Once the entire mixture is back in the pot, mix in remaining ingredients and serve garnished with parsley.

Simple and Scrumptious Potato Salad

This potato salad is super easy and healthy! Feel free to swap the additional vegetables depending on the season.

Vegetables
- 500g small red potatoes, peeled
- 2½ cups diced vegetables (e.g. capsicum, celery, red onion)

Sauce
- 1 cup raw cashews
- 1/3 cup water
- 1 tbsp olive or avocado oil
- 1 tbsp spicy mustard
- 2 tbsp white wine or apple cider vinegar
- 1-2 tbsp agave nectar or maple syrup
- 2 tbsp dried dill (or 4-5 tsp fresh)
- 1/4 tsp each sea salt & black pepper (plus more to taste)
- 3-4 cloves garlic (minced)
- 1 tsp hot sauce (optional)

For Serving (optional)
- Fresh chopped parsley

1. Add cashews to small bowl and cover with boiling hot water. Let sit uncovered for 1 hour.
2. In the meantime, add potatoes to a large saucepan and cover with room temperature water. Bring to a boil over high heat. Then reduce to medium-high heat so the water is at a low boil. Cook for 15-20 minutes or until tender and a knife easily slides in and out. Then drain and set on a cutting board or counter to cool slightly.

3. Once the cashews have soaked, drain well and add to a blender along with an additional 1/3 cup of water. Then add olive or avocado oil, wine or vinegar, spicy mustard, agave or maple syrup, dill, salt, pepper and garlic. Blend on high, scraping down sides as needed, until texture is creamy and thick but pourable. Add more water if needed for blending.
4. Taste and adjust flavour as needed, adding more dill for a herby flavour, garlic for zing/bite, salt and pepper for overall flavour, maple syrup for sweetness or vinegar for acidity. You can also add hot sauce for added spice (optional).
5. Chop cooked potatoes into bite-size pieces and add to a large mixing bowl along with chopped vegetables. Top with all of the sauce and stir to coat. Garnish with parsley (optional) and serve as is – slightly warm / room temperature, or cover, transfer to the fridge and chill until cold – 1-2 hours or overnight.
6. Leftovers can be kept in the fridge for up to 1 week, but are best eaten in first 72 hours.

DINNER

10-Minute Chickpea Curry

This is my go-to on a night when I get to 6pm and realise everyone is hungry and I haven't even thought about dinner. It's super quick, nutritious and so tasty!

Serves 4

- 1 chopped red or brown onion
- 1 tsp minced garlic
- 1 tsp minced ginger

- 1 tbsp curry powder (optional)
- 1 tsp paprika
- 1 tsp coriander
- 1 tsp cumin
- 1 can chopped tomatoes
- 1/2 can coconut milk
- 1 can chickpeas
- 1 tsp salt
- 1 tsp black pepper
- Lime juice

1. Heat water or oil in a pan over medium-high heat.
2. Sauté onion for a couple of minutes, then add garlic, ginger and spices.
3. Cook for another 2-3 minutes then add tomatoes and chickpeas.
4. Add remaining ingredients and let simmer for 10-15 minutes.

NB: This recipe can easily be bulked up by adding another 1-2 cans of legumes, such as black beans, red kidney beans, cannellini beans, etc. I also often cook a pack of gluten-free pasta then add it to the pot to bulk it up even further. Another option is to serve on top of cooked brown rice.

Comforting Creamy Pasta

Comfort food at its finest, but with much healthier ingredients! This is a firm favourite on the meal plans I give to my clients.

Serves 4

- 2 red onions
- 2 cloves garlic

Recipes

- 200g mushrooms (e.g. oyster, button, shiitake)
- 100g broccoli
- 2 tbsp tamari / gluten-free soy sauce
- 100ml vegetable stock or water
- 250g gluten-free penne pasta

Creamy Sauce
- 80g cashew nuts (roughly 10 nuts per person)
- 450ml non-dairy milk of choice (rice/ oat/almond/soy)
- Juice of ½ lemon
- 1 tsp salt
- 1 tsp garlic powder

1. You can roast the cashew nuts if you choose or use them raw. To roast, cook 5-8 minutes in a non-stick pan on medium heat. Be careful not to burn.
2. Peel and finely chop onions and garlic. Chop mushrooms and broccoli into bite-sized pieces.
3. Cook pasta as per instructions on the packet. Add broccoli so it cooks at the same time.
4. Drain and rinse pasta and broccoli once cooked to prevent further cooking.
5. Place a non-stick pan on high heat and allow pan to get hot. Then add onions and garlic and fry until they start to brown. Once they start to brown and stick, add 1 tsp of vegetable stock or water to clean the pan and incorporate browned flavour to the dish.
6. Add mushrooms and fry 2-3 minutes, adding a little water or stock if they start to stick.
7. Add 3 tbsp tamari/soy sauce and fry for a further 2 minutes. Turn off heat.

Creamy Sauce

- Blend all ingredients in a blender until smooth.
- Add pasta and broccoli to the mushrooms. Pour over creamy sauce (gradually so mixture doesn't end up too runny).

Buddha Bowl

Buddha bowls are one of my all-time favourite meals because they are so versatile, and you can put in whatever your heart desires! They are a great way to use up ingredients in the fridge or pantry. The general idea is to include a grain, a green, a protein and a healthy fat, but you can get creative and do what works for you.

Here's some ideas of what you can include:

- Veggies: Roasted veggies, leafy greens (kale, lettuce, spinach), chopped tomatoes, capsicum, cucumber, carrot, steamed broccoli/green beans
- Grains: Brown rice, quinoa, gnocchi, pasta, millet
- Proteins: Tofu, legumes, falafels, nuts, seeds
- Fats: Sliced avocado, pesto, nuts, seeds, olives
- Condiments: Salad dressing, hummus, homemade aioli dressing*

Start with the leafy greens at the bottom of the bowl, then layer the other ingredients on top and drizzle with homemade aioli or another dressing of choice.

*See recipe for aioli on page 196

Recipes

DESSERTS

Vanilla Chia Pudding

This pudding is so simple to throw together and tastes delicious. It can also double as a breakfast option.

Serves 1

- ½ cup almond milk, cashew milk or coconut milk
- 2 tbsp chia seeds
- 1 tsp maple syrup
- ½ tsp vanilla extract
- Fresh fruit, nuts and seeds

1. Add the chia seeds, milk, maple syrup and vanilla extract together in a bowl or jar and stir together. Let sit for 10 minutes, then stir again once the seeds have started to gel.
2. Cover the bowl or jar and place in the fridge for at least one hour. You can leave them overnight if you wish.
3. Stir the pudding before serving and add your favourite fresh fruit, nuts and seeds.

Decadent Chocolate Mousse

This decadent mousse is a favourite of mine. It also works well scooped into mini containers for school lunchboxes.

Makes 3-4 servings

- 1 can coconut milk or cream (full fat)

- ¼ cup cocoa or cacao powder
- 3-4 tbsp icing sugar
- ½ tsp pure vanilla extract (optional)
- 2-3 tbsp peanut butter (optional)

1. Refrigerate the coconut cream or milk overnight or freeze for 10 minutes. Try not to shake the can because you want the cream separate from the water underneath.
2. Once cold, open the can and transfer the thick part to a bowl. Use a beater to whip the cream until smooth.
3. Add remaining ingredients and whip it until it forms a mousse-like texture.

SNACKS

Berries and Cream

Here is a scrumptious morning or afternoon snack. Berries are a great fruit option because they are packed with antioxidants and healing properties.

Serves 2 to 3

- Up to 4 cups of assorted berries
- ½ cup of coconut cream
- 1 tsp grated ginger
- 1 tsp maple syrup
- 2-3 tbsp lemon juice
- Few drops of vanilla essence (optional)
- 1 tsp lemon zest
- 4 leaves of fresh mint (as a garnish)

Recipes

1. Divide the berries into two bowls.
2. Place the coconut cream into a mixing bowl.
3. Add the vanilla, maple syrup, ginger and the lemon juice.
4. Whisk until the mixture is smooth.
5. Top with lemon zest and mint and pour onto berries.

Fruit with Strawberry Drizzle

This is a great after-school snack for the kids to get involved in. The fruits below are just an example –use any seasonal fruits you like.

Makes 4 - 8 skewers

- 3 kiwis
- 1 cup berries of choice
- 2 bananas
- 1 cup dates
- 1 cup strawberries
- Splash of water if needed for the sauce

1. Combine the dates and strawberries in a blender and blend until smooth (you may need to add a splash of water).
2. Peel, slice and arrange the rest of the fruit on the skewers.
3. Drizzle the strawberry sauce over the skewers.

Baked Pears

A beautiful snack for a cold and wet day! You can use apples instead of pears if you like, and the recipe can double as a breakfast or dessert option.

Serves 2

- 2 pears
- 2 tsp maple syrup
- ¼ cup chopped walnuts
- ½ tsp cinnamon

1. Preheat the oven to 175 degrees Celsius.
2. Slice the pears length ways and remove seeds.
3. Place the pears face up in a roasting tray.
4. Brush with maple syrup over the face.
5. Divide the walnuts evenly across the pears and sprinkle cinnamon over the top.
6. Bake for 20 to 30 minutes.
7. If having for breakfast add some coconut yoghurt on the side.

SWEET TREATS

Chocolate Banana Poppers

I absolutely love these, and so do my kids. They are very easy to make and so yummy – not to mention healthy!

Makes several servings

- 4-5 bananas
- 1 block dark, dairy-free chocolate
- 2 tbsp smooth peanut butter (optional)

1. Melt the block of chocolate with the peanut butter (if using) in a glass dish over a saucepan of boiling water. Stir frequently until mixed together.

2. Place a whole banana in the chocolate mixture and roll it around until it's covered with chocolate.
3. Place chocolate-coated banana on a tray lined with baking paper.
4. Repeat with all the other bananas.
5. Freeze until solid, then cut into bite sized chunks.

Store in the fridge or freezer.

Chocolate Krispies

This is a great snack for the kids' lunchboxes because it's a definite treat, but without all the yucky stuff you find in the processed and packaged variety.

Makes several squares.

- 1 ½ cups smooth peanut butter (melt if necessary so it's easy to mix)
- 1 -2 tbsps extra peanut butter
- 1/3 cup maple syrup
- 1 tbsp vanilla essence
- 2 cups gluten-free rice pops
- 1 block dark, dairy-free chocolate (85% Lindt is a good option)

1. Mix together the first three ingredients then mix in the rice pops.
2. Pat the mixture into a greased or lined baking dish.
3. Melt together the block of chocolate and the peanut butter then spread over the top of the rice pop mixture.
4. Freeze for 30 minutes then cut into squares.
5. Store in fridge or freezer.

DRESSINGS

Aioli

This aioli recipe is so rich and creamy and a firm favourite in our fridge.

- 1 cup olive oil
- ½ cup unsweetened soy milk
- 2 cloves minced garlic
- 2 tsp lemon juice or apple cider vinegar
- ¼ tsp salt

1. Let the soy milk come to room temperature.
2. Add all ingredients into a blender and blend until thick and smooth.
3. Taste and adjust lemon juice or salt if required.
4. Store in the fridge for up to 5 days.

Peanut Sauce

A tasty dressing for a salad, to be used as a dip for fresh vegetables or for snacks such as tofu and spring rolls.

- 1 can unsweetened coconut milk (full-fat is best)
- ¼ cup Thai red curry paste
- ¾ cup natural peanut butter (or cashew butter or tahini)
- ½ tsp sea salt
- ¾ cup packed coconut sugar
- 2 tbsp apple cider vinegar or white wine vinegar
- ½ cup filtered water

Recipes

1. Combine all the ingredients in a medium saucepan. Place over medium heat and bring to a gentle boil, whisking constantly.
2. Reduce heat to low and simmer for 3-5 minutes. Remove from the heat and allow the sauce to cool and thicken.
3. Use immediately, or store in an airtight glass jar in the fridge for up to 2 weeks. The sauce will thicken in the fridge so you may need to add a little water before serving.

Digging up the Dirt

Where will you start with stocking your kitchen and which recipes will you try first?

Fabulously Full o' Beans!

Congratulations – you made it!

I know there's been a lot of information to digest and, like anything new, it can seem a bit overwhelming.

The best place to start is at the beginning, so my advice is to take a deep breath and start jotting down some notes about what that looks like for you. The questions I have set out for you at the conclusion of each chapter are designed for this very purpose – to help you get clear on where you're at now and how to take the first steps forward.

Will you start having a couple of meatless meals each week? Or using a plant-based milk in your tea or coffee? Will you make a more conscious effort to read nutritional labels or buy fewer packaged foods at the supermarket? Do you need to have a chat to your family about what kinds of meals you want to cook going forward?

Big changes don't have to happen overnight, so think about the ones that you want to try first. Sustainable, long-term changes come from doing things sensibly, so there's no point being a bull at a gate and then throwing it all down the gurgler when it seems too hard.

If you are really struggling with your health, I encourage you to transition towards a plant-based diet more quickly. I did this when I was very sick, and while it wasn't always easy, it gave my body the best chance to heal.

My hope is that this book has given you the background information and tools to get you started, and the knowledge about *why* you should start. As you would have seen with the testimonials and case studies, the WFPB is nothing short of life-changing and incredible results can happen with relatively little time and effort.

As always, I am here to guide you on the journey towards optimal health and wellbeing. I make the process super easy by providing you with meal plans, grocery lists and recipe books, along with everything else you need to know to make sure all functional pillars of health work in harmony.

Health must be your utmost priority for a long and vibrant life. There's no time like now to stop thinking and start doing.

Do you remember the promises I made you in Chapter One? Deciding to take action and making a commitment to your health means you are already 80% of the way there. The other 20% is in the action itself, answering the questions at the end of each chapter and following the tools and guidelines I have set out for you.

Fantastic health is our natural state of being and it's crucial if we want to live our absolute best life. We must rise above the challenges of the world around us and start taking full responsibility for our health.

The only person who can do this for you, is YOU.

So, what are you waiting for?

Now is the time for you to take the leap towards a whole-food, plant-based diet, experience for yourself the sensational benefits I've been promising you all along, and start feeling fabulously full o' beans!

About the Author

Heidi is the youngest of four children and was brought up on an orchard in Katikati, in the Bay of Plenty of New Zealand. After finishing high school, she gained a Bachelor of Arts, majoring in Japanese and International Business Management from the University of Waikato. The allure of travel and living abroad then led to a two-year OE in Japan and the UK.

After working in marketing and local government and seeking a new direction, Heidi completed a Diploma of Holistic Life Coaching through the Life Coach Associates of New Zealand in 2008.

During a health crisis in her late thirties that left her bedridden and disillusioned with conventional medicine, Heidi turned her focus to natural healing and gained a Certificate in Plant-Based Nutrition from Cornell University in the USA. From here, she joined her husband Steve in the family business, Jennings Holistic Health Coaching. Their vision is to transform the health and lives of 500,000 people around the world, with a safe and natural approach.

Heidi's ultimate goal is to educate and inspire those who are feeling defeated by their health, by showing them how the body can transition from surviving to thriving, given the right tools and support.

Heidi is the Amazon #1 Bestselling Author of *From Living Hell to Living Well*, a public speaker on the subject of health and wellness, and a freelance writer for national and global publications.

Today, Heidi lives in Tauranga, New Zealand, with her husband Steve, their daughter, Bonnie and son, Arie. In her spare time, Heidi loves to dance (Latin American) and go on long walks where she dreams up subject matter for future books.

Contact Heidi:

W: www.jenningshealthcoach.com
E: heidi@jenningshealthcoach.com
F: http://Bit.ly/HeidiJenningsPlantBased
F: http://Bit.ly/JenningsHolisticHealth

My Gifts to You

Personalised Coaching Opportunity

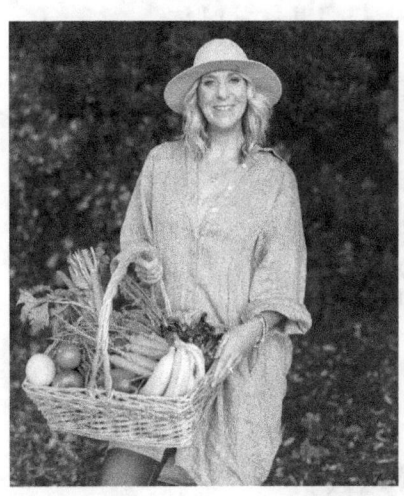

Are you struggling with poor health or feeling less than your best?

Are you fed up with a merry-go-round of pills and potions that don't work?

Are you ready to take charge of your heath and become the best version of you?

Secure a 30-minute Rapid Action session with a proven expert, who will help you map out a personalised path forward and revolutionise your health and wellbeing. If you're ready to experience vibrant health and vitality, this is a fantastic opportunity not to be missed. Quote *'Full o' Beans!'* to receive a 50% discount off your session. Be quick because spaces fill up fast!

Contact Heidi: *heidi@jenningshealthcoach.com*
www.jenningshealthcoach.com to secure your appointment.

Full o' Beans!

Free Starter Kit

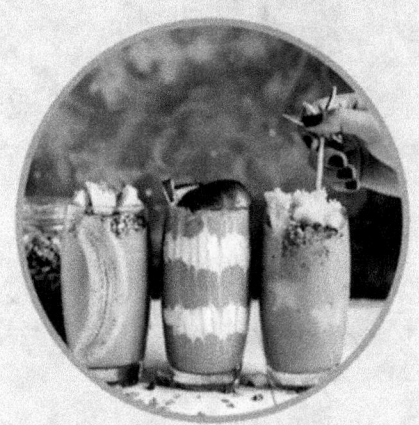

The Ultimate Five Steps to Functional Health

Learn the five pillars of optimal health and where to restore normal function

www.jenningshealthcoach.com

My Gifts to You

Do you feel stuck or frustrated about your state of health right now? Are you confused about how to get started on your path to wellness? Are you ready to take the first steps towards vibrant health?

Download our free e-book 'The Ultimate Five Steps to Functional Health' and identify where you need to take action right now with your health. Get clear on your motivation and reasons for change and take the first steps to completely transforming how you feel and show up in the world.

Download your copy at
www.jenningshealthcoach.com/fivefunctionalpillars

Full o' Beans!

Have You Read our Amazon #1 Bestseller Yet?

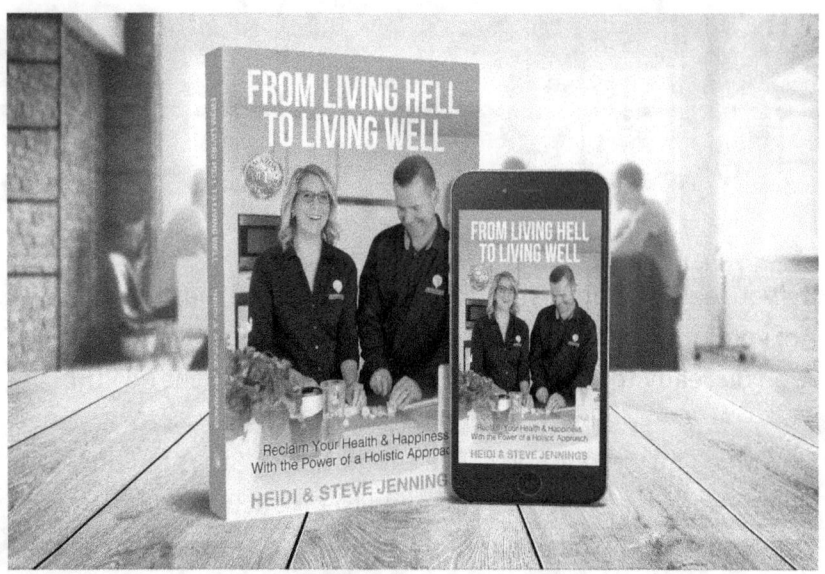

From Living Hell to Living Well

Are you stuck in a living hell with your health? Are you tired of going around in circles trying to find a solution?

Imagine being able to bounce out of bed in the morning with a clear head, an abundance of energy and a happy state of mind. Picture living inside a body that is the perfect weight for you and functions exactly as it should. Wouldn't you love to experience that kind of vibrant health and wellbeing, and the freedom it would bring?

The revolutionary blueprint for health developed by Heidi and Steve Jennings is the life-changing solution you've been searching for. Forget the pills, potions, fads and gimmicks that only lead to despair. Through the five pillars of health, you can experience the sublime state of being you deserve. It's straightforward, sensible and sustainable, and most importantly it actually works.

If you are suffering from chronic pain or inflammation, anxiety, depression, stubborn body fat, autoimmune dysfunction, menopause symptoms or sleep issues - or any other condition that lowers your quality of life and prevents you from being your best self - this book is a must-read for you.

It's time to put your hands back on the steering wheel, take control of your health, and live a life you truly love.

Available for purchase at *www.jenningshealthcoach.com*
Ebook available at *https://www.amazon.com/author/heidijennings*

Acknowledgements

Because the writing of this book came about rather quickly after publication of our first one, I must thank my husband Steve, and kids Bonnie and Arie for putting up with me tapping away on the keyboard furiously for long periods of time, yet again. Rest assured I don't intend to write a third book just yet – although that could change by next week.

To the Ultimate 48hr Author team – Nat, Stu, Julie, Vivi, Lendy, Nik and my editor, Alex, you guys are simply awesome, and I can't thank you enough for helping make my dream come true – twice!

Thank you to my ex-clients and case studies, Kylie Teague, Nola Darvill and Jenny for sharing your stories, I appreciate it.

A big thanks to my clients who know they need to take charge of their health and call on me to guide them through the process. It's such a privilege to work with you and I absolutely love seeing the changes that happen when you bring plant-based foods into your life. I can't think of a job more rewarding than the one I have, and I love every minute of it.

Thank you to the friends and family who support and encourage me to keep writing, particularly my parents, Anne and Harry Burggraaf.

Special thanks to Christine Norton, who once again kindly proof-read my manuscript.

Thanks to Amy Wolland for the awesome photo shoot where we nailed the perfect shot for the cover, and to Sita Sanders for working her magic beforehand!

Many thanks to Lynda Johnston who provided helpful guidance regarding content.

A massive thanks to Cornell University for providing an incredible course on plant-based nutrition and leading the way in this exciting field.

And thank you to you, my reader, for wanting to learn all about the plant-based lifestyle and trusting me to impart my knowledge and experience. May your newfound health and wellbeing take you wherever your heart desires to go!

Further Reading

The China Study, Dr T Colin Campbell
How Not to Die, Dr Michael Greger
UnDo it, Dr Dean Ornish and Anne Ornish
Your Body in Balance, Dr Neal Barnard
Prevent and Reverse Heart Disease, Dr Caldwell B Esselstyn Jr.

Further Viewing

What the Health
The Gamechangers
Forks over Knives
Seaspiracy
Cowspiracy

Heidi Jennings

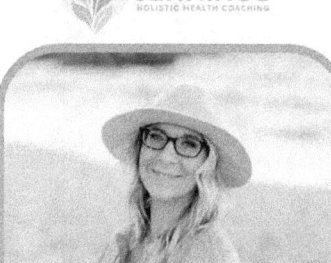

Holistic health coach and plant-based nutrition specialist Heidi Jennings is a sought-after leader in the health and wellness industry, who brings a wealth of knowledge and experience to her field. Her personal health transformation serves as an excellent foundation for helping her clients to overcome chronic health issues, with an impressive track record spanning hundreds of satisfied clients.

Heidi is the Amazon #1 bestselling author of *From Living Hell to Living Well* and has been featured in local and national media. She contributes to both domestic and global publications on the subject of health and wellness, and in 2021 she was selected as an official honoree for the BRAINZ Magazine Global CREA Awards for her contribution to mental health and leadership.

Heidi's ultimate mission is to spread her message and transform the health and lives of 500,000 around the world. She lives with her husband and two children in the Bay of Plenty, New Zealand.

Heidi can customise her key-note to any audience and time allotment. Her three signature talks are listed below.

Ultimate Blueprint for Optimal Health
- Take control of your health safely and naturally
- Supercharge the healing process
- Achieve life-changing, sustainable results in as little as six weeks

Transform Your Life with a Plant-Based Diet
- Why turning to nature can prevent and reverse disease
- Effective tools and strategies to ensure success
- Achieving your full potential through plants

Achieving Optimal Mental Health
- Uncover and address the root cause of stress
- Heal mental health conditions naturally
- How to fuel the body to fuel the brain

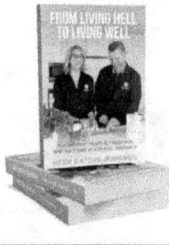
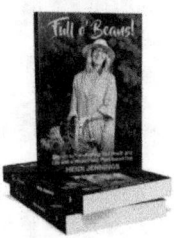

To enquire about engaging Heidi at your next event, email heidi@jenningshealthcoach.com or phone +64 21 0243 6217 for pricing and availability.

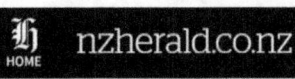
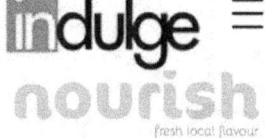
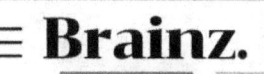

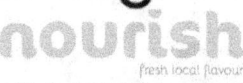
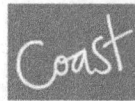
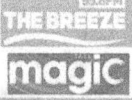

+64 21 0243 6217   heidi@jenningshealthcoach.com   jenningshealthcoach.com

Notes

Full o' Beans!

Notes